WHAT READERS SAY

"I have read and reread your most helpful book over the past ten healthful years (so have my significant others). The information was so helpful to me as a new diabetic. I am most thankful for the insight, humor, and honesty which you both offered in that book." M.S.

"Thank you so much for writing a book that is written to be understood by ordinary, everyday people." A.M.

"Your lighter, happy style has lifted my spirits immensely. If I can continue to approach the future with the attitude I have found in your writing, I *know* I will do OK!" P.N.

"First, I want to thank you for *The Diabetic's Book*. My husband was diagnosed with diabetes two weeks ago. All of the new information and change in life-style have been overwhelming; I can't tell you how many times we've picked up your book and found answers to our questions." S.S.

"Your writing soothes the soul while enriching your mind—and along the way gives a much-needed chuckle at just the right place. Thank you both." J.K.

"Recently I found out I have type 2 diabetes, and reading *The Diabetic's Book,* I thoroughly enjoyed the straight talk and the humor of it. I feel I am more aware of how I can cope with the everyday life of diabetes. Hats off to June and Barbara!" B.B.

"I am seventy-seven years old and am insulin dependent. I have your book *The Diabetic's Book* and it is almost a second Bible to me. Thanks for the help I've gained from it." Mrs. R.M.

THE DIABETIC'S BOOK

ALSO BY JUNE BIERMANN AND
BARBARA TOOHEY

The Peripatetic Diabetic

The Diabetic's Sports and Exercise Book

The Diabetic's Total Health Book

The Diabetic Woman (with Lois
Jovanovic-Peterson, M.D.)

The Diabetic Man (with Peter Lodewick, M.D.)

Psyching Out Diabetes (with Richard R.
Rubin, Ph.D.)

Diabetes Type II and What to Do (with Virginia
Valentine, R.N., C.D.E.)

The Diabetes Sports and Exercise Book (with Claudia
Graham, C.D.E., Ph.D., M.P.H.)

JUNE BIERMANN AND

BARBARA TOOHEY

T H E

Diabetic's Book

·*all your questions answered*·

Jeremy P. Tarcher/Putnam
a member of Penguin Putnam Inc.
New York

Most Tarcher/Putnam books are available at special quantity discounts for bulk purchases for sales promotions, premiums, fund-raising, and educational needs. Special books or book excerpts also can be created to fit specific needs. For details, write or telephone Putnam Special Markets, 200 Madison Avenue, New York, NY 10016; (212) 951-8891.

Jeremy P. Tarcher/Putnam
a member of
Penguin Putnam Inc.
200 Madison Avenue
New York, NY 10016
www.penguinputnam.com

Library of Congress Cataloging-in-Publication Data

Biermann, June.
The diabetic's book: all your questions answered / June Biermann and Barbara Toohey. — 4th ed.
p. cm.
Includes index.
ISBN 0-87477-924-3
1. Diabetes—Miscellanea. I. Toohey, Barbara. II. Title.
RC660.B459 1998 98-4630 CIP
616.4'62—dc21

In memory of
JACKIE TIPPEN
who for thirty-five years
gave us the two greatest gifts:
love and work

Contents

All things are difficult
before they are easy.

—THOMAS FULLER, 1608–1661
Gnomologia No. 560

Foreword

An old Talmudic saying goes, "All beginnings are difficult." This couldn't be more true for persons with diabetes. To begin life over as a diabetic person is not only difficult but slightly short of impossible. Receiving the diagnosis of diabetes has nearly the same jolt as seeing your whole life—your inner house—collapse after an earthquake or hurricane.

The Diabetic's Book: All Your Questions Answered can be your guide to that new beginning. June and Barbara will lead you through the rebuilding and healing process with sound advice, knowledge, and wisdom gained over many years. They take the guilt out of "getting" the disease. It is hard to move forward when fear, anxiety, and anger are all pushing you back. Diabetes self-care necessitates information, skill, and concentration. This book provides it all.

Let me tell you why I feel so strongly about this tome.

First, it truly answers all your questions, as the title suggests. I know of few other books on diabetes that contain the wealth of information you will find here. The advice and facts are not only up-to-date but are substantiated by an extensive literature review and the secondary opinions of many leading experts in the field of diabetes self-care. June and Barbara also give you their own firsthand experiences and those of many other real people who live with diabetes day in and day out.

Second, this book teaches you the basic language of diabetes in a clear and straightforward manner. Each and every time a medical term is used, it is explained and defined. This is no small feat. One of the worst complications of diabetes is actually the misunderstandings that frequently occur between diabetic patients and their health care team. Thus, your new language skill will mean that the important communication between you and your doctor and dietitian can begin.

Third, this work speaks to every diabetic, regardless of whether you are type 1 or type 2 (you will learn the difference in the first section), young or old, in control or out of control. I am particularly pleased with the coverage June and Barbara have provided for the person with type 2 diabetes, who is so often forgotten in other books on diabetes. In the past, type 2 diabetes was thought to be a mild disorder that did not demand attention to blood-glucose control. Today, we now know that type 2 diabetes needs the full respect that the type 1 diabetes always had. Those of you with type 2 diabetes need to keep your blood-glucose levels as near to normal as possible to avoid the complications of diabetes. To achieve this goal, the type 2 diabetic must adhere to diet, medication, exercise, and blood-sugar monitoring. This change in the philosophy of type 2 diabetes treatment and self-care is clearly explained and beautifully chronicled by June and Barbara.

Fourth, there is a level of detail in this book that is unmatched in other beginner diabetes manuals. In every section, Barbara and June provide tiny gems of information that one generally does not find elsewhere. From diet tips to exercise hints to insulin injection equipment to advice for parents and families, you will find dozens of ideas that can truly make life easier for all involved.

From their suggestions, I learned to watch business trends for the latest breakthrough developments in diabetes control and treatment. Barbara and June are so right about this. After all, it only makes sense that we will learn about new discoveries and inventions in the pages of *The Wall Street Journal* and other business magazines before new diabetes products hit the market. By staying abreast of the business news, every diabetic person can follow the research done at dozens of companies and thereby feel a bit more hopeful that a cure is on the way.

Lastly, and perhaps most important, this book will motivate you to make the necessary changes in your life to live well with diabetes. As you read these pages, I am sure you will feel, as I did, that you are in good hands and that you have been truly understood. Through their own experiences with diabetes, Barbara and June know the ins and outs of depression, frustration, and fear. They write sensitively about what every diabetic person and concerned family member goes through, and they teach you how to have a sense of humor about it. It is easier to laugh when you know you are not alone, and diabetes is so much more tolerable to live with when you can laugh about dietary restrictions, injections, blood tests, mood swings, and annoying itches. June and Barbara will almost make you feel sorry for persons who do not have diabetes!

You will also find that this book can motivate your family and friends to a new beginning as well. The section addressed to them is worth the price of the book alone. Not only will they start to understand your diabetes, but they will gain a new sense of themselves and the role they can play in helping you to live a full and satisfied life rather than, as often happens, making "your" problem "their" problem.

When you have finished reading these pages, I am sure you will agree with my sentiments about this wonderful book. Thank you, June and Barbara. I enjoyed, I learned, I identified with all you have to offer here. Bravo for your new edition of *The Diabetic's Book*. All my questions *were* answered.

Lois Jovanovic-Peterson, M.D.
Director and Chief Scientific Officer,
Sansum Medical Research Foundation,
Santa Barbara, California
Clinical Professor of Medicine,
University of Southern California,
Los Angeles

THE DIABETIC'S BOOK

Introduction

Although this book is intended for anyone involved with diabetes—whether a newly diagnosed or experienced diabetic, a family member or friend, or a diabetes health professional—it is aimed primarily at beginners.

Why beginners? For two reasons. The first was born one day when the June half of our writing team was emerging from her dentist's office. The door to a neighboring internist's office opened and a man came out. He was clutching a copy of the American Diabetes Association's approved diet guide, *Exchange Lists for Meal Planning.*

The man had obviously just been given *the news,* because in ninety-six-point headlines his face was printed with confusion, fear, and despair. June could read these emotions easily because they were the same ones she'd seen in the mirror on her own D (for *diagnosis*) day. While writing this book, we've kept this man's face before us. Our goal has been to change his expression—and that of all newly diagnosed diabetics—to one of understanding, courage, and hope.

The second reason for aiming this book at beginners is based on the Zen theory of the expert's mind versus the beginner's mind. Since the expert's mind thinks it knows everything, it is closed to new ideas. It knows what *can't* be done. It thinks in terms of limitations. The beginner's mind, on the other hand, is still open. To the beginner all things are possible. Not even the sky is the limit.

We hope that this book will help all of you—no matter how many years you've had diabetes or have worked in the field of diabetes—to become beginners again.

THE DIABETICIZATION OF AMERICA

Lonely and lost though you may feel at the time of diagnosis, you are not alone in your diabetes. In the sixteen years since the original publication of *The Diabetic's Book,* America has been what you might call "diabeticized." The estimated number of diabetics has risen from 10 million to over 16 million, and about a third of these are undiagnosed. As the population ages and longevity increases, the incidence of diabetes correspondingly goes up. The financial impact of this escalation of diabetes is $138 billion a year. In June 1997 new effort was launched to ferret out more undiagnosed people and get them into treatment, thereby reducing the human and medical costs of the serious complications of diabetes. The participants in this effort—several health agencies, including the American Diabetes Association and the Centers for Disease Control and Prevention—announced new recommendations for implementing early diagnosis. They advised that everyone over the age of forty-five should get a blood test to check for diabetes at least once every three years, and those above 20 percent of their ideal weight should do so more often. These new guidelines mean that diabetes will get more and more serious attention; consequently, people with this disease will receive improved therapies and care. In conjunction with this development, in August 1997 President Clinton "unveiled a plan to battle diabetes," as the newspaper headlines put it. He announced that the federal government would spend $2.1 billion over the next five years for diabetes treatment and research. Now that's more like it!

Consider the contrast with the way things were back in 1967

when June was diagnosed. Although it was not the worst of times, it certainly was not the best of times. Practical help for those with diabetes ranged between scarce and nonexistent. The now active, ten-thousand-member American Association of Diabetes Educators didn't even exist. The available diabetes books were ponderous and discouraging and written in boring, incomprehensible medical language. Those greatest tools for keeping your blood sugar under control—home blood-sugar-testing meters—hadn't been invented. People with diabetes were condemned to use inaccurate, awkward, and distasteful urine tests. Blood-sugar tests were given monthly or quarterly, even in some cases annually, in the doctor's office.

Because of this lack of help, information, and effective technology, we started devoting ourselves to finding ways to cope successfully with diabetes without becoming a slave to it and giving up all joys and excitements.

Using June as a guinea pig, we constantly checked out new angles of attack, seeing just how far we could push the envelope of diabetes. In conversations after our talks at diabetes associations, and in correspondence with hundreds of other diabetic people and health professionals who shared our good-life goals, we continued to learn more. We have shared this newfound, ever-expanding, and changing store of information and experiences in ten previous books on diabetes—including the three previous editions of this one.

Because *The Diabetic's Book* is our most basic and accessible book on diabetes, and because it has been used as a teaching text in many diabetes education programs, it has been read by more people than any of our other books on the subject. Over 150,000 copies are out there somewhere in Diabetesland. It has made us happy to be able to reach and, we hope, *teach* so many of those involved with diabetes. But a cloud slips over this happiness when we realize that a lot of the material from the last edition has already become out-of-date.

You'd think that in only four years not enough of significance in the field of diabetes could happen to warrant a fourth edition. But, believe us, it has! Nothing makes us more jubilant than to be able to tell you that so many changes for the better and so many breakthroughs have come about in this four-year period that this rewrite is mandatory. We don't want any of you to miss out on the new knowledge and therapies to make your life easier, happier, healthier, and *longer*. You'll find it all in this newly revised edition.

All in all, if you had to become diabetic, this is the best time in the history of the world for it to happen. Never before has it been so possible to keep your blood sugar in the normal range, to avoid (or reverse) the feared complications of diabetes, and to enjoy life as it was meant to be enjoyed. With this book we want you to learn how to live better with diabetes and *through* diabetes.

June Biermann
Barbara Toohey
Van Nuys, California
January 1998

Something for Everyone

The old saying "You can't see the forest for the trees" is, like many such sayings, very insightful. Sometimes you're so close to the individual aspects of a problem, you can't see the whole picture. And not seeing the whole picture may prevent you from gaining the perspective necessary to attain overall control of the situation.

Therefore, before we launch into the specifics of how to take care of yourself as an insulin-taking or non-insulin-taking diabetic, or how to master the emotional aspects of the disease and manage your daily life, or how to offer the best support possible for your diabetic family member or friend, we'll take a look at the big picture of diabetes. This is what everyone needs to know. You'll find that once you see the forest of diabetes, you'll find it easier to get out of the woods.

DIABETES AND CONTROL

What is diabetes?

Diabetes is a physical problem that causes you to have too much sugar in your blood. The medical name for it is *diabetes mellitus*. The Latin word *diabetes* means "siphon," and *mellitus* means "honeysweet." The two words together are usually translated "sweet water siphon." (In case you don't speak Latin, *diabetes mellitus* is pronounced *dye-uh-**beet**-ease **mell**-uh-tus*.) The doctors in ancient times called it that because they noticed that diabetics urinated a great deal and that their urine tasted sweet. Yes, *tasted* sweet. In those days the only way a doctor could test urine was by tasting it. (And doctors today won't even make house calls!)

In June 1997 at the American Diabetes Association 57th Scientific Sessions, a committee of experts from various health agencies (the Expert Committee on the Diagnosis and Classification of Diabetes Mellitus) set up new classifications of diabetes. This was the first revision since 1979. Maybe you've heard of the old terms insulin-dependent diabetes, called Type I, and non-insulin-dependent diabetes, called Type II. The experts no longer think these names useful and instead they recommend just using the terms "type 1" and "type 2." You'll notice that, to avoid confusion, they've dropped the Roman numerals in favor of Arabic. Although we confess to a certain nostalgia for the Roman numerals we've used for over thirty years, we've capitulated and gone Arabic throughout this book.

Virginia Valentine, R.N., C.D.E., our friend and collaborator on *Diabetes Type II* [*sic*] *and What to Do,* says wryly of the new classifications, "New names, new numbers, same damned disease." Indeed, the expert committee's definitions do have a familiar ring:

> In type 1 diabetes your body destroys the cells in the pancreas that produce insulin, usually leading to a total failure to produce insulin. It typically starts in children or young adults who are slim, but can start at any age. It afflicts about 700,000 Americans. In type 2 diabetes the body cannot use insulin properly and sometimes doesn't produce enough insulin. It usually occurs in people over forty-five and overweight among other factors. About 7 to 7.5 million Americans have been diagnosed and another 8 million remain undiagnosed with type 2 diabetes.

Though these are the two main types of diabetes, there is yet another, which—unlike the other types—is not ordinarily permanent. It's called gestational diabetes and only occurs during pregnancy. The 1997 expert committee describes it as follows: "A condition of abnormal glucose metabolism that arises during pregnancy, gestational diabetes complicates about two to four percent of all U.S. pregnancies. Although it usually disappears after birth [of the baby], gestational diabetes may signal an increased risk for type 2 later in life."

In all types of diabetes the basic problem is that without treatment there is too much sugar in the blood.

Why is there too much sugar in the blood?

The cells of the body run on a fuel called *glucose*. This is the sugar that the body manufactures from the food we eat. Glucose is carried to the cells in the bloodstream, but if you have diabetes it cannot be absorbed because the cells are locked up tighter than a Manhattan apartment. Glucose can't get into a cell without a key. That key is *insulin*. Insulin is a hormone that comes from a gland called the pancreas. The particular cells of the pancreas that produce insulin are the beta cells.

In type 1 diabetes the beta cells have been totally destroyed and make no insulin, or have been partially destroyed and don't make enough insulin. That is to say, all or some of the insulin keys are missing, so they can't let the sugar into the cells. Such people will need to inject insulin—we will explain that later.

In type 2 diabetes the beta cells are still there perking along, manufacturing plenty of insulin keys, but either the cells in the bloodstream don't have enough locks (called insulin receptors) for the insulin key to fit in, or something is keeping the locks from working. (This is called insulin resistance or insulin insensitivity.) These people need to modify their diet, lose weight, and make other changes to control their diabetes. We will also explain this treatment shortly.

In both cases, the result is that sugar is left in the bloodstream, causing high blood sugar.

There is a convenient test doctors use to determine whether a diabetic still makes any insulin and roughly how much. It is called a C-peptide test and is a blood test ordinarily taken after overnight fasting and before breakfast. The more insulin your body makes, the higher your C-peptide level. The level of blood-serum C-peptide is usually zero in type 1 diabetics. In type 2's it can be within or above or below the normal range.

What's wrong with having high blood sugar?

High blood sugar is an indication that your body is getting little or no fuel. In desperation it begins to convert its own fat and muscle into fuel. This is like chopping down the walls of your house to get wood to burn in your fireplace. If you keep that up, soon you have no house left.

But that's not even the worst of it. When the body burns itself for fuel, excess *ketones* (substances that are formed during the digestion of fat) are given off. These excess ketones can poison the body. This poisoning—called *ketoacidosis*—can lead to death. You may remember the television program about the California boy, Wesley Parker, whose father threw away his insulin because a faith healer had "cured" the boy's disease. Within three days Wesley was dead from ketoacidosis.

There is also something else wrong with having high blood sugar. Let's say you have *some* insulin that's working—either insulin you've injected or insulin you've produced in your own pancreas—but you don't have enough. Or say you have plenty of insulin, but it's not able to get the sugar into the cells. Then, while you won't use up your own body as fuel, and you won't be poisoning yourself with ketones, you still have too much sugar flowing through your bloodstream. That's not good, because this situation brings about long-range diabetes complications like blindness, nerve damage, kidney failure, and gangrene of the feet.

What caused me to get diabetes?

Researchers have been puzzling over the answer to this question for decades. They have more leads now than ever before but still no definitive answer. We'll summarize what is known, and you can apply the information to yourself.

First, diabetes runs in families; so whether you got it as a child or later in life, you still had to have some genes that predisposed you to it. The two different types of diabetes are caused by different genes. Type 1 is much less hereditary than type 2. Second, diabetes favors certain ethnic groups: the incidence in African Americans, Hispanics, Native Americans, and Asians is much greater than in the Anglo population.

If you got type 1 diabetes as a child (the commonest age to be diagnosed is around twelve) recent studies show that a virus related to the mumps, measles, or a similar infection might have attacked the insulin-producing beta cells of your pancreas. This triggered an immune response, so that your body's own immune system continued the destruction until after several years your insulin-producing capability was totally gone and you had diabetes. One study suggested that drinking cow's milk as an infant might trigger this same response. Scientists also suspect a possible environmental factor in childhood diabetes, since the highest incidence occurs in cold climates, and more cases are diagnosed in winter than in summer.

For those diagnosed in midlife or later, the type 2's, more than one genetic defect is responsible. This form of diabetes develops slowly over a period of years. Before most adults are diagnosed with type 2 diabetes, they often have gone seven years or more with the disease. The number one factor influencing the appearance of diabetes is excess weight. Some 80 to 85 percent of those diagnosed are overweight. Another influence is aging and a general slowing of body functions. More cases of diabetes are diagnosed after the age of fifty than at any other time of life.

Oddly, physicians have also discovered a special form of type 2 diabetes that affects children and young people under the age of twenty-five. This is called MODY (maturity-onset diabetes of the young). Like adults, the children diagnosed with MODY are usually very overweight.

Overproduction of certain hormones—growth hormone from the pituitary, thyroid hormone, epinephrine, cortisone, and glucagon—makes the body's insulin less effective and can also bring on diabetes.

Pregnancy, which makes additional demands on the body, can cause diabetes to develop. In fact, some women show diabetes symptoms during pregnancy, but their symptoms disappear after the baby is delivered. (This is called gestational diabetes.) Mary Tyler Moore wasn't that lucky. Her diabetes was diagnosed shortly after a miscarriage, and since then she has been insulin-dependent.

Surgery or a major illness can activate diabetes. June became diabetic not long after a hysterectomy.

Many people have the mistaken idea that they can get diabetes from eating too much sugar. (Diabetes is sometimes called "sugar diabetes," which adds to the confusion.) Diabetes can't be caused by eating too much sugar, except when your diabetes was triggered by overweight and you became overweight partly from overloading on sugar. But even in that case, it wasn't specifically the sugar that was to blame. Diabetes could have developed if you ate too much of anything and gained weight. The culprit is more likely the fat in your diet.

Why didn't I have any symptoms of diabetes when my case was diagnosed?

You were one of the thousands of hidden diabetics—people who have diabetes and don't realize it. You're one of the smart (or lucky) ones. You caught diabetes early, before it had done any real damage.

If you neglect your diabetes in the future, you may begin to experience the classic symptoms of the acute stages of diabetes: excessive urination and thirst, increased appetite, rapid loss of weight, irritability, weakness, fatigue, nausea, and vomiting. These indicate ketoacidosis, which if untreated will lead to coma and ultimately death. These are the symptoms that usually strike children and adolescents suddenly.

Most people who get type 2 diabetes after the age of twenty have a different set of symptoms, though they may also have any of the above. Generally, the warning signals are drowsiness, itching, blurred vision, tingling and numbness in the feet, fatigue, skin infections, and slow healing. Type 2 diabetics often have two additional clues that diabetes may be in the offing: they are overweight, and they have a family history of diabetes.

Can my diabetes be cured?

In the last edition of this book we said, "Things are looking up. Scientists are working on a number of possibilities." This is still true, but we appear to be stuck in the realm of possibilities. Scientists are working on many of the same solutions and some exciting new ones, but we still can't announce any definitive results. Our counsel is to take good care of yourself, keep your diabetes under control, remain optimistic and hopeful, and be expectant of one of those medical miracles that occur these days with increasing frequency. Then when the cure *does* come, you'll be in good shape and ready for it.

Among the possibilities researchers are currently exploring are:

ISLET CELL TRANSPLANTATION

Transplantation of the islet cells of the pancreas that produce insulin is still being investigated, as it has been for twenty years, but few experiments are taking place now in the United States because of a government moratorium on the use of fetal tissue. The major technique under trial is to encapsulate the cells in a porous membrane (like plastic) that would have large enough pores to let insulin out but would be too small to let the body's immune system in to attack the transplanted cells.

PANCREAS TRANSPLANTATION

Since 1978 over two hundred transplants have been done in the United States. If the pancreas alone is transplanted, the success rate is only 60 percent, but this increases to 75 percent when both the kidney and the pancreas are transplanted at the same time. The scarcity of pancreases available for transplantation means this cure is available to very few people.

IMMUNIZATION

The current emphasis is to prevent diabetes in those who have a strong family history of it. Presently it is possible to test such people for antibodies and determine whether they are on the road to type 1 diabetes. A study currently under way, called the Diabetes Prevention Trial, Type 1, is screening large numbers of people who fall into the high-risk category. These people are then given low doses of insulin to prevent the destruction of their beta cells.

A Diabetes Prevention Program for type 2 is also under way. It will identify those at high risk and try different strategies to prevent insulin resistance. Some people will receive counseling in diet and exercise; others will be given oral hypoglycemic pills or a placebo. Results of both these investigations won't be ready until 2002.

The American Diabetes Association (ADA) recently set new standards of blood-sugar levels by which to identify people at risk for diabetes. The diagnosis of diabetes is now to be made on the basis of a fasting blood-sugar level of over 126. Previously the cutoff point was 140. This means more people will be moved in to the diagnosed category and will begin treatment early enough to prevent or delay the complications of diabetes.

Studies to identify the gene of inheritance for both types of diabetes are also being conducted. The hope is that in the future people can be immunized against diabetes just as they are against smallpox and polio.

How can I avoid the complications of diabetes?

We have mixed emotions about ranting at you about diabetes complications. Some doctors and nurses feel that unless they paint vivid horror pictures, diabetics won't take their disease seriously and do what they should to take care of it.

Sometimes this backfires, though, as we learned in a letter from one diabetic. On the first day of her diagnosis and hospitalization, she was told by the head nurse, "You have a dreadful, dreadful, dreadful disease." The nurse convinced her that all she had to look forward to was "becoming a blind, bilateral amputee, carried off to dialysis three times a week." This experience so affected her psychologically, she wrote, that

> I lay awake night after night shaken with an unbearable fear. It permeated every aspect of my daily life. I gave up wearing contact lenses because I cried so much. I was worn out emotionally. My college doctor suggested psychiatric counseling. I was hesitant, but after six months I was helped greatly and started taking better care of myself because I finally felt there was a glimmer of hope for the future.

On the other hand, we can't just ignore or gloss over the complications. They can happen, but you have it in your power to make them *not* happen by keeping your diabetes under control—that is to say, keeping your blood sugar normal most of the time.

Many people involved with diabetes, either as patients or health professionals, have long believed that it's possible to avoid complications by keeping blood sugar in or near the normal range. As diabetic diabetologist Richard K. Bernstein, M.D., stated years ago, "Diabetes doesn't cause complications; poor therapy causes complications."

But still there has been an ongoing debate on the subject. Despite the anecdotal evidence and passionate proselytizing by those of us who were True Believers in tight control, many health professionals remained unconvinced. They were unwilling to impose a more rigorous regimen on their patients without incontrovertible scientific proof that the effort would pay off.

Now the doubters are convinced, thanks to the Diabetes Control and Complications Trial (DCCT), which gave scientific proof that good control can prevent—and in some cases reverse—diabetes complications. The DCCT was conducted at twenty-nine American and Canadian medical centers. Over a ten-year period it followed 1,441 people with type 1 diabetes. The patients in the study were divided between those using the "conventional" diabetes treatment of taking only one or two shots of insulin a day and one blood-sugar test and those using a more "intensive treatment." This intensive treatment involved taking three or four shots of insulin (or using an insulin pump that continuously delivers small amounts of insulin) and doing a minimum of four blood-sugar tests a day. Even though the blood-sugar levels of those using intensive treatment were still somewhat above those of nondiabetics, they were much closer to normal than those using conventional therapy. The mean daily blood sugar of the intensive group was 155; that of the conventional group was 231.

Dr. Orville Kolterman, head of the University of California, San Diego, test site, called the conclusions of the study "fairly spectacular." And so they were. Diabetic retinopathy was reduced by 76 percent, kidney disease was prevented or delayed by 56 percent, and neuropathy (nerve damage) by 60 percent. Since the study groups were relatively young (ages thirteen to thirty-nine) and in relatively good health, there were not enough cardiovascular incidents to prove that the intensive treatment would be of help in preventing those, but one of the doctors in charge said that even in that area "the trends are very encouraging."

But how about people with type 2 diabetes? Does tight control help them as well? The ADA in their Position Statement say that it's not known for certain, but they conclude that it seems reasonable to recommend tight control in many type 2 patients since it is presumed that the cause of complications would be the same in both types.

The morning after the results of the study were made public, Mary Tyler Moore, who was on a more conventional therapy for her diabetes, appeared on *Good Morning America*. When asked if the study might cause her to change to a more intensive therapy, she responded, "I'm changing today!"

The interviewer asked her if she'd had any complications besides the retinopathy for which she'd received successful laser treatments. She said she didn't think so, but added, "Diabetes is like a great-looking house that has termites. You never know what's going on in there."

Good control is like tenting and fumigating that house and getting a lifetime guarantee that the termites are gone.

How do I keep my blood sugar normal?

You asked the question correctly: "How do *I* keep my blood sugar normal?" Because diabetes is the original do-it-yourself disease. Although you'll have help and guidance from the health professionals on your diabetes team, the responsibility for day-to-day therapy is all yours.

Normalizing blood sugar involves many aspects of your life and life-style. You need a good diet, preferably one tailored to your needs by a dietitian, a sound exercise plan that you can stick to, some stress-control techniques that appeal to you and work for you, and self-education with magazines, books, and lectures to keep your knowledge growing. That will about do it for the great majority of you. Some type 2 people will need to take pills, and some will need insulin. All type 1 people will need insulin.

Now we come to the key question of what normal blood sugar is. The normal range is around 60 to 140 milligrams of sugar per deciliter of blood. (Milligrams per deciliter is usually abbreviated to mg/dl.) We think the objective of most all diabetes treatment should be to keep blood sugar within this range; in other words, in tighter control than in the DCCT study. Ideally, each person's goals should be set individually. As was stated when the DCCT results were announced, "No formulas can be applied to every patient and therefore intensive therapy must be used with prudence and common sense." This caution applies especially to people with heart problems, the elderly, and those type 1's subject to sudden, severe attacks of low blood sugar. They may be advised for safety's sake to keep blood sugars in higher ranges.

After you eat, your blood sugar rises and reaches its peak between a half hour and one hour later. In nondiabetics it rarely goes over 140. Blood sugars above 160 suggest that a person is diabetic. Here is the normal pattern of blood sugar for nondiabetics in relationship to meals:

RELATION TO FOOD	BLOOD-SUGAR RANGE
Fasting (before breakfast)	60–100
1 hour after meal	100–140
2 hours after meal	80–120
3 hours after meal	60–100

Diana Guthrie, a professor of nursing at the University of Kansas School of Medicine in Wichita, has provided us with this chart of recommended blood sugars for diabetics.

RELATION TO FOOD	IDEAL	ACCEPTABLE
Fasting	70–110	60–120
1 hour after meal	90–150	80–180
2 hours after meal	80–130	70–150
Pre-meal or 3 hours after meal	60–110	60–130

You'll notice that on these charts the blood sugars you should aim for have both a lower boundary and an upper one. Although diabetes is primarily associated with blood sugars that are too high, insulin-taking diabetics often run the risk of having blood sugar that is too low. Low blood sugar, known as hypoglycemia, can result from too much insulin, too little food, too much exercise, etc. We will go into the details of hypoglycemia in the section for insulin-dependent diabetics. Type 2 diabetics who take pills can sometimes experience hypoglycemia, but it is milder and less frequent. We'll discuss that in the section for type 2 diabetics.

Can anything besides eating and not eating make my blood sugar go up or down?

Yes, and you need to take these factors into account. Blood sugar often goes up when you have an infection—the flu, the common cold, stomach upsets. Major surgery and pregnancy cause a rise. Then there are a number of drugs that tend to raise blood sugar: caffeine, oral contraceptives, estrogen, and cortisone are the most important to know about. Emotional tension also causes blood sugar to swing upward.

Besides being lowered by fasting or by insufficient food, blood sugar goes down when you exercise strenuously. Among drugs with a lowering effect are alcohol (when you don't eat while drinking), large doses of aspirin, blood-thinning drugs, barbiturates, and sulfonamides.

For a complete list of medications that increase or lower blood-sugar levels, see the first page of the reference section.

How will I know if my therapy is working?

You take tests. Most of your testing will be self-testing. In a sense, you are your own laboratory technician. Here are the tests you will learn to perform or have performed.

Blood-sugar test. Your most important and most frequent test is a blood-sugar test. Only by testing your own blood sugar can you tell from day to day how well your therapy is working. And only if you make a record of your test results can your doctor see how good your control is or what modifications in your treatment are needed to improve it.

Thanks to modern technology, self-blood-sugar testing, called "monitoring," is getting faster and more trouble-free. Your results are available in between ten seconds and two minutes, depending on the system you're using. Blood-sugar testing is performed by putting a small drop of your blood on a pad. Then you compare the color that the pad turns to a color chart (the less expensive method) or you use an electronic meter to interpret the blood sugar from the pad and give you a digital readout. This is more expensive but more accurate. Some of the newer meters use an electronic sensor rather than a chemically treated pad.

Most diabetes health professionals consider the development of self-blood-sugar testing to be the greatest advance in diabetes treatment since the discovery of insulin in 1922. Everyone should take advantage of it.

Type 1 diabetics typically need before-meal and after-meal tests, before-exercise and before-driving-a-car tests, and tests whenever they feel symptoms of low blood sugar. Almost all type 2's need tests before breakfast (fasting) and some one-hour-after-meals tests. Those on medication (pills or insulin) need before-breakfast and before-supper tests plus some after-meals tests.

Granted, this kind of careful self-care means using a lot of those expensive testing strips. If finances are a problem, there is one thrift measure you can take, but you'll have to settle for the less accurate visual testing. You can cut Chemstrips bG in half lengthwise, thereby getting two tests for the price of one. Plus you'll have the additional advantage of using a smaller drop of blood. (If you determine your insulin dose by your blood-sugar test, visual testing is not recommended.)

Hemoglobin A_1C test. Another test for assessment of control that all diabetics should use is the hemoglobin A_1C test, also called the glycosylated hemoglobin test. This test, combined with daily blood-sugar readings, gives you a total picture of your diabetes control, as it provides you with the long-range view.

An A_1C test should be taken about every three months. The A_1C

test is a laboratory test that is taken in your doctor's office. It analyzes how much glucose (blood sugar) has bonded with your red blood cells. This measurement indicates what your average blood sugar has been over the past eight to ten weeks. The A$_1$C test aligns closely with risks for diabetes complications. That's why it's important to have it taken about every three months.

The Becton-Dickinson Company has announced that their at-home A$_1$C test will be available in 1998 at a cost of $20–$30. You stick your finger and place two drops of blood on a specially treated test strip that is sent to a lab in a prepared mailer. You and your doctor will then receive the test results by mail within seven to ten days. For more information, contact Becton-Dickinson at 1-800-237-4554.

Fructosamine test. The fructosamine test is a glycated protein test just like the A$_1$C. Both tests indicate the average blood-glucose levels over a prior time frame, but they measure different time frames. While A$_1$C measures glucose control over the prior two to three months, fructosamine measures a much tighter window, just the prior two to three weeks. Fructosamine tests are particularly useful for type 2's who only take a limited number of blood-glucose tests or for people who are sunable or unwilling to follow a daily testing program. Fructosamine tests are also valuable for all those who want to keep close track of their treatment plans. The *Johns Hopkins Guide to Diabetes for Today and Tomorrow* also suggests that they can provide useful information "if it's desirable to get a short-term average—for example, during a pregnancy."

A new at-home meter system that performs the fructosamine test, also called the GlucoProtein test, has been released by the LXN Corporation of San Diego, California. It's called the Duet meter, because it can perform blood-sugar tests as well as the fructosamine test. It's a sort of all-in-one system with two different kinds of strips: Duet test strips for blood glucose and GlucoProtein test strips for fructosamine. For information, call 1-888-596-8378.

Urine test. Before blood-sugar testing came on the scene, urine testing was the only way we had to know how well our diabetes was being controlled on a day-to-day basis. When blood sugar goes too far above normal, usually 150 to 180, some of the sugar spills over into the urine so that the body can get rid of it. Measuring the amount of sugar in your urine was supposed to indicate your blood-sugar level, but it was very inaccurate because:

- it indicated only what your blood sugar had been, not what your blood sugar was at the time of the test;
- it couldn't tell you if your blood sugar was too low (hypoglycemia);
- it could be affected by such things as the amount of water you'd been drinking and any vitamins you'd been taking; and
- not everyone spills sugar when their blood sugar is between 150 and 180. Older people often don't spill until it's much higher (June doesn't spill until she's over 220), and children can show sugar in their urine when it's lower than 150.

So our advice is to forget urine testing except when you need to test for ketones.

Ketone test. You'll remember that ketones are the substances that can accumulate in the blood in uncontrolled type 1 diabetes or in uncontrolled type 2 diabetes when there has been total loss of insulin production by the pancreas. They indicate an insufficiency of insulin, and, as we pointed out earlier, the body begins burning its own muscle and fat for fuel. Ketones are the by-product of burning body fat as an energy source. They cause a toxic acid accumulation in the blood that leads to what is called ketoacidosis or DKA. DKA can lead rapidly to coma and death. It is a medical emergency of highest concern.

If, on the other hand, you have well-controlled blood sugars but are on a low-carbohydrate weight-loss program, ketones will indicate that your diet is successful because you're burning your own fat. Unlike ketoacidosis, mild ketones in this case are not dangerous. They are the normal result of the low-carbohydrate weight-loss diets to be discussed later.

How do I test for ketones?

A better question might be, *When* do I test for ketones? The answer for type 1 diabetics is whenever two consecutive blood-sugar tests are over 250. For type 2 diabetics who still produce insulin of their own, the situation is not so crucial, but all diabetics need to watch for ketones when they have infections, illnesses, or out-of-the-ordinary emotional stress.

The brand-name products to use for urinary ketone tests are Chemstrips uGK, Chemstrips K, Ketostix, and Keto-Diastix.

What's the most accurate blood-sugar meter?

This is the foremost question asked about meters. In truth, all meters function well and have acceptable accuracy. The Food and Drug Administration (FDA) must approve a new meter before it's released to the public. Since most meter studies are financed by a meter company and their meter invariably comes out on top, we'd never seen an unbiased meter rating report until *Consumer Reports* came up with one in their October 1996 issue. At that time there were twenty-one different models on the market, and they tested only eight of the leading ones—those manufactured by Bayer, Boehringer-Mannheim, Lifescan, and Medisense. They reported, "All meters we tested provided results that were accurate enough to be used with confidence." The Glucometer Elite (Bayer) was rated number one for convenience, consistency, and accuracy, and the One Touch (Lifescan) was a close second. But then was then, and now is now. The meter scene is so constantly changing, with "new and improved meters" appearing almost monthly, that no meter can stay number one for long, and none is ever selected as the best by all reviewers.

If you have a meter made by an established company, you don't have to worry about its accuracy. If you want to worry about something, worry about your competency in using the meter. That's what really counts. That's why all meter manufacturers continually try to make their instruments as operator-independent (a nicer way of saying fool-proof) as possible: "No buttons, no wiping, no blotting, no timing, no cleaning," etc. They realize that ease of use leads to accuracy. Then, along with the need for competency, there's the psychological aspect of blood-sugar testing. When people report that a meter is inaccurate, what many of them really should be saying is, "I don't like what this meter is saying about my blood sugar, so it must be wrong." The technical services department of one meter company once reported that 90 percent of the meters returned to the company as reading inaccurately were operating perfectly.

How do I select the meter I can operate most accurately?

The answer is simple: Select the one your doctor or diabetes educator recommends. This is a good idea for several reasons. It is usually the meter they use in their own office. It will therefore be easy for them to check out your meter (and your technique) any time you come into the office. Having the same meter as your health professional will give both of you confidence in the accuracy of your own test results. Health professionals have their prejudices, too. They often think the meter they have—and are most familiar with—is the only truly accurate meter.

Some doctors also have a machine that prints out your blood-sugar readings from a specific meter. In that case, they'd want you to have the meter that's compatible with their machine. Be sure you find out *exactly* which meter they recommend before you go shopping. Have them write down the name for you, because meter names are very similar, and it's easy to get them confused.

If your health professional has no particular preference, you need to find the meter that's best suited to your life-style, economic situation, manual dexterity, visual acuity, blood volume, and aesthetic taste and to find out whether the strips for the meter are covered by your health plan. To figure out all this, you'll need to read *Diabetes Forecast*'s annual "Buyer's Guide to Diabetes Supplies" (the October issue) and check the brochures of those of interest to you or, better still, see all the meters in person and have someone knowledgeable explain the features of each. That kind of service is very rare these days, because there are now so many meters, each company spinning out a new version every year or so, that no diabetes center or supply house can make them all available or afford such a large instructional staff. For that reason you need to use almost as much care in selecting where you buy the meter as in selecting the meter itself.

Where should I get my meter?

Try to find a diabetes supply outlet or teaching center or pharmacy that will give you personal instruction in operating the instrument. This is particularly important for those who have never taken their own blood sugar, not even with a visual strip. First-timers must learn how to get a drop of blood from a finger stick and apply it to a test strip. This maneuver requires a very special technique for each type of strip. Strips come in all sizes and forms. Some are foil-wrapped and not easy to open. Some are tricky to load into the meter. Some require much more blood than others. Some absorb blood easily, while with others it wants to skate off. Even if you have to pay more for the meter, get as detailed a lesson as you can, including having your instructor watch you perform a sample test and critique your technique. Go back for a second training session if you feel insecure.

How much should I pay?

Meters run the gamut in the sophistication of their technology and in their cost. Depending on how basic or advanced the meter is, where you buy it, and whether you pay or have the outlet bill your insurance, pricing goes from free or under $50 (often with a rebate and/or trade-in) up to around $100 (with kits that provide all essential supplies).

In buying a meter, remember, the meter itself is a one-time expense; what you really need to consider most is the price of the strips that are used with it. Each year they go up, all of them in lockstep. Some are as high as 80 cents each.

Our philosophy is to buy the meter you're most happy with if you can possibly afford it. A meter you find compatible with your skills and life-style is a great bargain compared to a cheap one you'll leave on a shelf to gather dust.

The final essential consideration is the customer service and reliability of the company that manufactures the meter. The best companies offer total support: an 800 telephone number, twenty-four-hour customer service staffed by polite and knowledgeable personnel, overnight replacement of ailing meters, help and advice with operational problems. And you need a company that's large enough to have wide distribution of its strips so that you aren't locked into buying them at very few outlets. A meter with limited strip availability is a handicap and a hassle.

It's a nice dividend if the place that sells you the meter will also handle your insurance claims, but if your choice is between a place that gives good instruction and doesn't make claims and a mail-order company or pharmacy that does, you're better off choosing the instruction and making the claims yourself, unless your insurer doesn't let you.

How can I be a smart shopper?

The lowest prices on meters, strips, and all other supplies are from the mail-order companies that advertise in *Diabetes Forecast* and other magazines and newsletters. The convenience is great, too, because you don't have to drive there, park, and stand in line. But there are lots of bewares on this subject.

Since they don't give instruction, buy a meter by mail order only if you're an experienced operator who's upgrading and can learn from a manual, a tape, or a video (some companies supply free training videos). And be sure to order supplies far enough in advance so that you won't run out before the next shipment arrives. Also, always check the expiration date on test strips and make sure you can use them all before the deadline.

The smart shopper doesn't just worry about price. He or she takes great pains to learn the brand names of every item used with the meter. Otherwise, on your first shopping trip to replenish supplies you'll run into a lot of trouble. You may end up with the wrong product and not be able to return it if you opened it. And the brand names of all diabetes supplies are often confusingly similar. Our advice is to take along your empty containers or write down the names of the supplies you need and take the list with you.

How can I know my meter is delivering correct results?

It's only human to worry about the accuracy of your meter—especially when it gives you a number you don't like or can't explain. After all, you're using the meter to guide you through your therapy, and you want to make certain it's not sending you off in the wrong direction. But some people go too far with their suspicions. They get to the point that they spend more time and effort fiddling and fretting with their meter, taking it back for a replacement or a totally different meter, than they do actually testing their blood sugar and figuring out how to improve their therapy to get better results.

Human though this "inaccurate meter syndrome" may be, you should try to avoid it. It's far better to regard your meter as a friend who wants to help you rather than an enemy out to thwart you. Here's a little self-analysis that may help you build a better and more productive relationship with your meter.

- Are your expectations of the accuracy of meters beyond their present capability? We find that people have a mistaken notion of the preciseness of meter readings. Meters give you a *range* of correctness, not one figure that represents your absolutely correct and specific blood sugar at that moment. If you get a number within 10 or 15 percent of your actual blood sugar, that's great. That's all you need to know for good control. Take that figure and adjust your food, exercise, or medication according to your doctor's guidelines.
- How is your technique? Many of the inaccuracies in meter results are due to operator error. You might want to go to your doctor or diabetes educator or the place where you purchased your meter for a review lesson and technique check.
- How clean is your meter? A dirty meter is an inaccurate meter. You should have a regular meter-cleaning schedule and also clean it anytime it looks as if it needs it. (Cleaning is not a problem with certain new meters that use an electronic sensor that extends out from the meter so blood never touches the machine itself.)
- Do you want a way to verify that your meter is functioning properly? Use the control solution that comes with your meter—or buy new if it's out-of-date—and test your meter with that. (Hospitals do this every morning. Or at least they're supposed to!) These solutions have a preset glucose level. Some companies have them for normal, low, and high ranges. If your control test falls within the range printed on the solution insert, then your meter is A-OK. Don't be surprised at the broad range considered acceptable. It may be something like 88–123 or 85–157.
- Does your test result make absolutely no sense to you? Then do a second test and see if it comes out near the first or tells you something different that you can believe. If the second test falls

within the same ballpark and you're still dubious, buy some Chemstrips bG and do a visual test. A visual test is mainly good for checking if you're very high or very low, but even so it can help you settle your controversy with your meter. (Incidentally, it's not a bad idea to keep visual strips around in case your meter goes completely bonkers or kaput or you drop it and break it or take it somewhere and lose it.)

• Are you truly upset and desperate? Call the 800 number of the meter manufacturer and see if they can help you ascertain if your reading was correct. Besides, it will give you some relief just to explain your problem to someone and maybe yell a little bit.

A final piece of advice for everyone about meter results. Whenever you go to the doctor's office and have a blood-sugar test taken there (they always want to do their own), take your meter and do a test yourself the moment after they finish. If your result comes within 10 or 15 percent of theirs, you'll go home at a good comfort level with your meter. Warning 1: Don't take your blood sugar at home before you go to the doctor and expect it to be the same as the test in the doctor's office. That's how many people start developing the "inaccurate meter syndrome." The passage of time and the stress of being in a doctor's office can make dramatic differences in your blood sugar. Warning 2: If there's a great discrepancy between the reading on the doctor's meter or lab test and your meter, it could be that yours is right and theirs is wrong. Stranger things have happened.

What can I do if I have trouble getting enough blood for the test?

First, try to relax. When you're tense, your blood tends to leave your extremities and go to your body organs to prepare you for the fight-or-flight response. You can tell if you are relaxed if you have warm hands.

Then make sure you're using the correct tip for your lancing device. Some of them have a choice of tips, one with a larger opening that makes a little deeper penetration than the normal tip. There is also the Auto-Lancet, which has a tip that adjusts with five settings to match your skin type. If you've checked that out and still have trouble, try some (or all) of the following:

1. Wash your hands with soap and very warm water. Allow warm water to run over your hands and wrists for at least one full minute. (Be sure you dry your hands thoroughly before starting your test.) Incidentally, washing your hands is much preferable to cleaning with alcohol. Not only does alcohol, when used repeatedly, dry out your skin, but if it hasn't evaporated before you take your test it can change the reading you get—usually making it lower.

2. Let your hand hang loosely by your side and shake it for at least thirty seconds.

3. Keeping your hand below heart level, milk the palm of your hand all the way up to the fingertip. Make sure the fingertip turns pink.

4. Prick the meaty side of the finger—not too close to the cuticle but not directly in the center (pad) of the finger or at the very top of the fingertip.

5. Allow your finger to relax for three to four full seconds before trying to squeeze the blood out. When you're cut or stuck with a sharp object, the muscles tighten up to prevent the release of blood. After a few seconds they relax and the blood flows easily again.

6. Milk your finger, starting with the base on the palm side and working all the way up to the fingertip. Wait two or three seconds between milkings.

How do I keep a record of my blood-sugar readings?

It's great that you realize you should keep track of your blood-sugar readings. Blood-sugar testing is not an end in itself. You don't just test your blood sugar, look at the result, and say, "Nice test, there" or "Rotten test there," and go about your business. The results of your tests are important information to give health professionals so that they can analyze and evaluate them to see if your control can be improved. If you don't keep accurate records, they can't do the best job for you. The records are also valuable to you in seeing patterns in control—and lack of control.

Many blood-sugar monitors now have memories ranging from one test all the way up to 300. But even if you're using a meter with a memory, you need to write down your test results in a log book so they can be quickly viewed and assessed from the point of view of deviations from your target ranges. Most meter companies provide one log book with the initial kit, but after you fill that one you have to keep buying them (usually for around $1 each).

Incidentally, if you enter all your blood-sugar tests in your log book, you can then add them up periodically and calculate your average blood sugar. Oddly enough, this correlates very well with an A_1C test. That is to say, if your average falls within the normal scope (70–140), you would probably come out in the nondiabetic range on an A_1C test also. And doing an average is a heckuva bargain compared to $40 for an A_1C lab test plus a doctor's office visit. In *The Diabetes Self-Care Method,* Drs. Peterson and Jovanovic-Peterson explain that if you take a measurement before each meal and a second one about an hour after you've eaten, the sum of the six tests should add up to about 600, and that gives you an average blood glucose of 100. Perfect!

How can I learn more about taking care of my diabetes?

Read books. Read periodicals like *Diabetes Forecast, Diabetes Self-Management, Diabetes Interview,* and *Diabetic Reader* (see the list of magazines in the reference section).

Join your local affiliate of the ADA (see the directory of organizations in the reference section) and attend their meetings. They usually have guest speakers—podiatrists, dietitians, ophthalmologists, or other professionals—who can fill you in on their own areas of expertise and answer questions that may have been puzzling you. Diabetes associations often sponsor day-long seminars with different speakers, panel discussions, and workshops. These are a terrific way to get a lot of diabetes information in a short period of time.

Find a diabetes education program in your area. Ask the ADA for names and places, or write to the American Association of Diabetes Educators (AADE) (see the directory of organizations in the reference section). These education programs sometimes charge a nominal fee, but you always get a lot more than your money's worth.

Diabetes education programs can involve a one-week crash course or weekly meetings over a period of time. They can be inpatient programs for newly diagnosed diabetics in the hospital, but most are outpatient. They can involve large or small groups, or they can offer individual instruction. There may be a group of teachers (nurses, dietitians, psychologists, social workers, etc.) or there may be one diabetes educator who handles the whole course. As you can see, you can usually find a program to meet your needs, whatever those needs may be.

Another way to learn is from other people with diabetes by sharing helpful information, experiences, and mutual concerns. There are over eight hundred diabetes support groups in the United States. Our favorite psychologist, Dr. Richard Rubin, tells us of the benefits of such a group. "The good ones help people feel less isolated, more comfortable with their diabetes, and more able to do the right thing when it comes to their self-care. In addition, support groups are free or, at most, require a small contribution. That's a real benefit. I encourage people to join support groups. Look for one you like and keep looking until you find one."

Ask your doctor and your diabetes educator and call the closest ADA and Juvenile Diabetes Foundation offices to find a group. If you can't find one, start one yourself. And how do you do that? You ask someone who has done it successfully, like Bettie Norgord, founding mother of the Dynamic Sharpshooters, a group that in ten years has grown to 425 members. For advice and counsel, contact Bettie Norgord, 4677 W. Earhart Way, Chandler, AZ 85226 (Phone: 602-940-9377).

If there is no support group in your area and if you're a computer nerd—as we are—you can surf for support on the Internet. For example, on America On Line, go to Channels, click on Health and then click on Support Groups and then click on Diabetes, Thyroid, and other Endocrine Disorders Support Groups. There you will find the location of support groups and their meeting time. Another route to take from Health is Illnesses and Treatments. When you click on that, you'll find a whole bunch of clickables for specific areas of diabetes information (for example, Gestational Diabetes, Diabetes Eye Disease, Organizations and General Information, etc.). Click and ye shall find. Also see Diabetes Web Sites in the reference section.

Where can I find out about the latest developments in diabetes therapy as soon as they happen?

You could read diabetes publications. But a surer method is to keep track of the *business* of diabetes. Business magazines and newspapers like *The Wall Street Journal* often beat the *Journal of the American Medical Association (JAMA)* and the *New England Journal of Medicine* in announcing new diabetes products. Better still, ask a stockbroker to send you prospectuses of companies involved in diabetes research, equipment, and products.

As an illustration, we read in the *New York Times* "Business Day" (November 17, 1997) that Amylin Pharmaceuticals of San Diego, California, has developed what their PR people call "the first new diabetes drug since the discovery of insulin in 1921." The patent they've just filed is for a synthetic version of a natural hormone called amylin, which was discovered about ten years ago. This hormone circulates in the blood alongside insulin, and acts to slow the inflow of glucose into the blood.

It works in tandem with insulin so that you're controlling the inflow of glucose as well as the outflow. The new drug, called Pramlintide, promises to make the use of insulin more predictable and lead to better blood-sugar control. Amylin Pharmaceuticals will be requesting FDA approval in the year 2000.

Not to discount altruism, but considering the growing diabetic population, it's not surprising that many companies are entering the field with big-time profits in mind. But whyever the developments occur, we'll be happy just so long as they do occur and make diabetes therapy easier and better.

Cautionary note: Most new drugs or technologies don't work even though they seem promising at the outset. So when you read about spectacular new products that sound like just what you need, don't let your hopes—or your investment dollars—get out of hand.

DIABETES AND YOUR EMOTIONS

How can I keep from being depressed over my diabetes?

It's not easy. It's only logical to be depressed when you first learn you have diabetes. And all the cheerful remarks people make about how much nicer it is to have diabetes than leprosy or than being run over by a moving van or some such nonsense do no good at all. You know that it's *not* better than having nothing wrong with you.

After all, you have to make many, many changes in your life, and at first glance these changes all seem to be for the bad. On top of that, you feel like an outcast. You're no longer like everyone else. Of course, no one ever *is* like everyone else, but at the moment you feel like the town pariah, and you're certain that all your friends are going to drop you now that you have diabetes.

You get the automatic "Why me?" reaction. "Why should *I* be selected to get this rotten disease?" "Why should *I* be threatened with blindness or kidney failure or gangrene or an early death if I don't fol-low a rigid regimen?" Why indeed? There's really no reason. It's just the breaks of the genetic game. As a doctor told us once at a meeting, "Every person carries around about forty-four genetic defects." One of yours happens to be diabetes, and the fact is that some people draw out far worse tickets than diabetes in the genetic lottery. But that doesn't make you feel any better. As A. E. Housman said, "Little is the luck I've had / and, oh, 'tis comfort small, / to think that many another lad / has had no luck at all."

So what do you do about all this? You can sit and resentfully mut-ter about cruel fate and wallow in your woe, or you can, as the old say-ing has it, take the lemon you were handed and make lemonade out of it. We read an article about a woman who is a successful author and consumer advocate on radio and TV in Los Angeles. She described her beginnings: "When we married, during the early years it was rough. We were poor, but I wasn't about to go on welfare. So I decided if I wanted clothes, I had to make them. If I wanted the best bread I'd better learn how to bake. What I did was take poverty and turn it into an art."

What you need to do is take diabetes and turn it into an art. Do all the things you need to do for your diabetes and make them en-hancements to your life.

How do I turn diabetes into an art?

The beginning step is to accept the fact that you have diabetes. The first thing most people do with diabetes is to deny it. Oh, your mind may know you have diabetes, but everything else about you—your heart, in-nards, soul, imagination, all those things you really listen to—say, "This has nothing to do with me. I'll ignore it and it will go away."

Alas, it won't, and you'll never be able to practice the art of dia-betes until you get rid of the idea you don't have it. As a matter of fact, you need to do more than just accept your diabetes. One young woman, after hearing us speak at a diabetes meeting, said to June, "You actually seem to embrace diabetes." That she does. Not that she wouldn't prefer not to have diabetes, but since she does have it, she's determined to squeeze all the good out of it she can.

What's good about having diabetes?

Without being ridiculously Pollyannaish about it, we can affirm that diabetes *does* do some positive things for you. This isn't just our idea. Many diabetics have written to us and told us about what they consider to be the advantages of diabetes.

For one thing, you learn the principles of good health. Until you're whammed with something dramatic like diabetes, you may just bumble along wrecking your health through bad habits, laziness, and ignorance. Diabetes teaches you the right way to live and gives you a reason for doing so. As one diabetic skier put it, "This disease, this condition will keep you healthy and fit for whatever your heart desires."

Diabetics often actually feel better than they did before having their disease. Young diabetics have reported to us that they do better in sports than their nondiabetic friends because they never eat junk food and always keep regular hours. They're in top-notch shape all the time. Professional motorcycle racer Michael Hunter says unequivocally, "If I didn't have diabetes, I wouldn't be as good as I am." Well-controlled diabetics also say they're less susceptible to colds and flus that their friends pick up with seasonal regularity.

Diabetics often look better than their nondiabetic contemporaries. Conscientious diabetics are lean and vital, bright of eye and quick of step. People of the same age who don't have diabetes to goad them onto the path of healthful living are often pudgy, sallow, and lethargic.

Diabetes develops self-discipline. Young persons who have diabetes and must assume responsibility for their own care develop a mature attitude of self-sufficiency at an early age. The discipline of following the diabetic way of life carries over to school and work and sports and creative endeavors. It can help make you a successful person in all areas of living.

Sometimes diabetes even sparks ambition. We know a young diabetic woman who is a successful city attorney. She told us how her choice of a profession came about: "When I got diabetes in high school I knew I'd have it all the rest of my life. I realized it would be an expensive disease, and I decided I wanted to always be able to take care of myself—and take care of myself *well*—whether I ever got married or not. That's why I worked hard to prepare myself for a good career."

And having diabetes makes you more compassionate toward others with problems. You learn how to give help gracefully and receive help without embarrassment or resentment. This, after all, is what puts the humanity in human beings.

But perhaps best of all, diabetes makes you capable of change. To change is the hardest thing for people to do. That's why so many of us take the easy way out and stick in a rut for our entire lives, unable to rouse ourselves into action to make the changes that could make us into the persons we were meant to be.

Diabetes, because it requires changes, and rather dramatic changes at that, shows you that you *can* change. If you can change in one area, then you are capable of change in other areas. You can improve not only your health but your whole life.

How do I start making all the changes I have to for my diabetes?

You phrased that correctly. *You* have to make the changes. As psychologist Dr. Richard R. Rubin said in *Psyching Out Diabetes,* "No one can make anyone else do anything." Try as they may, health professionals and concerned family members and friends can't force you to make the changes your diabetes requires. And they certainly can't do it for you. It's all up to you.

As we said before, your first step is to wholeheartedly acknowledge that you have diabetes and that it's here to stay. That gets you halfway to change land. The next step is to—as the new psych jargon puts it—*empower* yourself: realize that you *can* control your diabetes and your health and your life. Now you're three-quarters there. All that's left for you is to make those changes.

At this critical point we often hear the plaint, "I just can't get my-self motivated to _____ (exercise, test my blood sugar, lose weight, change my diet, etc.)." What will get you over the motivation hurdle into change? Dr. Rubin says it can be something positive like falling in love, wanting to have a baby, or becoming a grandparent. Or it can be something negative like the first harbingers of a complication. But you're buying high-priced trouble if you wait around until fate brings you a wonderful positive motivator or you start feeling the first twinges of neuropathy. It is far better to motivate yourself as did a young woman from Hawaii who wrote to us.

Motivation is the reason I'm writing. Your book deals with the diabetic who can't seem to get motivated. I've also heard this from diabetics I've met in Hawaii who are still feeling sorry for themselves rather than doing something. My mo-tivation is quite simple. I look down at my two feet and thank God they are at-tached to two legs. I also thank God that my eyes function so I can see those feet. I want to keep my feet and keep my eyes. THAT is motivation. As much as I love food, there is no food tempting enough for me to give up my feet or my eyes. So whenever temptation comes along, I just look down at my feet.

Those feet can make that important final step into change.

But so much of the change seems to be giving up pleasures. How can I feel good about that?

We found that when June, in her early fits of depression, was ticking off all the pleasures she'd have to give up because of diabetes, what she was really ticking off were habits. Something like eating a sweet dessert was a habit that she considered a pleasure merely because she'd done it so often that it was a comforting part of her daily routine. The trick is to establish new *good* habits and turn them by constant use into pleasures.

This is not as hard as you may think. Eating a delectable, juicy piece of fresh fruit can become as much of a habit-pleasure as eating a big, gloppy dessert. For many people a daily bike ride or after-dinner walk is a pleasurable habit, and it can become one for you, too.

Furthermore, when you're thinking of the things you have to give up because of diabetes, think of these: You have to give up ever waking up with a hangover, either of the cigarette or alcohol variety; you have to give up discovering on a shopping trip that you've ballooned another dress or suit size; and you have to give up feeling and looking like a couch potato because of lack of exercise.

Finally, if, as you make the changes in your life, you still have moments of depression, try to keep in mind that it's part of the human condition to be depressed from time to time. There will be a natural tendency for you to lay your every woe on the doorstep of your diabetes. That's unfair to diabetes. Bad though it may be, it's not enough of a villain to be responsible for every dismal moment in your life. Even if you didn't have diabetes, you wouldn't be frisking around in a constant state of ecstasy. Though they call life the human comedy, it isn't all laughs for anybody.

But it isn't all tears, either, and you should make every effort to emphasize the good aspects of your life—to make yourself into a happy person.

How do I make myself happy?

You just do it. As Mark Twain said, "Everyone is just about as happy as he makes up his mind to be." And Robert Louis Stevenson believed that "there is no duty we so much underrate as the duty of being happy." So make up you min .nd do your duty. It's vital that you do so for an important reason.

Not that you need a reason to justify happiness. It's a perfectly wonderful end in itself. But the reason we have in mind has only recently come to light. Studies reported in the *New York Times* show that being a happy, good-natured person can make you healthier, and that being an angry, suspicious person can be literally lethal: "People who are chronically hostile, who see the world through a lens of suspicion and cynicism, are particularly vulnerable to heart disease."

But that's not all. According to Dr. Ray H. Rosenman, a cardiologist at the SRI International Research Institute, hostile people are more prone to die prematurely from *all* causes, including cancer. They even get minor ailments like colds and the flu more often than happier people.

Your anger doesn't have to be the explosive, blow-your-top variety, either; more subtle styles of hostility—skepticism, mistrust, a tendency to make snide comments—are just as damaging. Strangely enough, even competitive, hard-driving type-A personalities who are not hostile are less at risk than their more antagonistic counterparts.

Try this experiment. The next time you feel hostile and angry, take your blood sugar. Assuming your negative feelings aren't due to low blood sugar, you'll probably discover your blood sugar ascending. Conversely, when you feel happy, take it and you may find, as June did once when she was looking forward to a trip to San Francisco, "I'm so happy I can't keep my blood sugar up."

Another reason to try to cut back on your anger is because of what it does to those around you. Many diabetics are angry because they have diabetes, but they don't like to admit the source of their anger, not even to themselves, so they displace their anger onto something or someone else. It could be the doctor's bill or the meter that gives a high blood-sugar reading or the health professional who's trying to help them make changes in their lives that they don't want to make or even their loving family members and friends.

The worst thing about displaced anger is that if you never admit its true source, you'll never get rid of it. It will keep festering within and erupting without.

Even if you acknowledge that your anger is diabetes-related, how do you deal with it? Dr. Richard Rubin explains that anger is "a signal that something is wrong, that you're feeling vulnerable, scared, hurt, embarrassed, attacked or overwhelmed. This causes you to react in one of three ways: (1) passively by burying your feelings, (2) aggressively by lashing out with anger, or (3) assertively by dealing straightforwardly with the situation." *Psyching Out Diabetes,* a book we wrote with Dr. Rubin, shows how to handle anger assertively, as well as how to rid yourself of other negative emotions like depression, fear, and frustration that cloud your existence and block out the sunshine of your life. (For more on this book, see the reference section.)

How does getting emotionally upset affect my diabetes?

An emotional upset has about the same effect on blood sugar as chocolate-chip cookies. A fight with an intimate, a boost in rent, a week of final examinations—any stressful event in your life can send diabetes dramatically out of control. The strange thing is that even if something favorable takes place in your life, that, too, can sometimes raise your blood sugar. When we were consultants on a tour to Hawaii for diabetics, several of the participants told us they got out of control with the excitement of packing for the trip.

Our own experience has convinced us that if you're working very hard at good control and usually achieve it but find that during certain periods there is a change for the worse and you can't figure out why, try getting out from under your normal life situation, especially if it's more hectic than usual. You may find, as June frequently does, that there's nothing wrong with your diabetes therapy, but that there *is* something wrong with your life and that *that's* what needs to be changed.

We are so convinced of the need for diabetics to learn how to handle the stresses of contemporary life that we wrote an entire book on the theme. The revised edition of *The Diabetic's Total Health Book* explains why tensions and stresses have a negative effect on diabetes, what stressors you can avoid, and how to develop techniques to keep those you can't avoid from upsetting your control. A good portion of that book is devoted to instruction in relaxation therapies. These therapies—exercise, self-hypnosis, biofeedback, meditation, and guided imagery—are the best preventive medicine ever invented. Each of you should start practicing the ones that appeal to you most. You'll particularly enjoy practicing our unique all-purpose relaxers: laughter, travel, pets, and hugs, all of which will enhance your life and the lives of all those around you.

For a clincher to a winning attitude toward life, you might read "Good Times Therapy" at the end of *Psyching Out Diabetes* (1997 updated edition).

DIABETES AND YOUR DIET

What is the diabetic diet?

This is no longer a simple question to answer. Years ago everyone was condemned to the same rigid little one-sheet list of permitted foods known as the diabetic diet. It was boring and limited with no accounting for individual tastes or ethnic preferences and, worst of all, seemed to ignore completely that the ideal diet for each person is the one that best meets two criteria: (1) it keeps the person's blood sugar normal, and (2) he or she enjoys eating it.

Over the last decades dietary recommendations have evolved and changed, but the basic eating plan has always been geared to the *Exchange Lists for Meal Planning* of the ADA and the American Dietetic Association. These lists divide food into six groups of similar foods (starch/bread, meat, vegetables, fruit, milk, and fat). You're assigned a certain number of choices (exchanges) from each list for each meal. This makes it easy to plan meals of great variety yet similar nutritional content.

In 1994 the ADA issued its new dietary guidelines, a dramatic breakthrough from the past. Diabetic eating was simplified and liberalized to the point that even the age-old taboo against sugar was removed. For example, under the new guidelines, a tablespoon of sugar can be exchanged for half a cup of mashed potatoes because each is one starch/bread exchange. But you can guess which choice nutritionists consider preferable. Furthermore, the ADA revised its one-size-fits-all standard advice about the proportion of carbohydrate, protein, and fat allowed in the diet. (All foods are composed of various percentages of these three nutrients.) Formerly, the proportions recommended on a per-meal basis were 55 to 60 percent carbohydrate, 12 to 20 percent protein, and 20 to 30 percent fat. Now you are to eat 10 to 20 percent of your calories in protein and divide the remaining 80 to 90 percent between fats and carbohydrates, depending on your own weight concerns and particular health risks such as cholesterol and triglycerides. The amount of carbohydrate you eat is more important than the kind.

At last, as you can see, your diet can now be individualized and your meal plan tailored to your type of diabetes, weight, exercise pattern, life circumstances, and personal taste. This means your diabetes diet can be adjusted to you rather than your having to adjust to it.

We consider the ADA formulas and exchanges, especially since they're now so much more flexible, a viable middle path to dietary planning. They're not, however, the only choice or necessarily the way for everyone to go. There are advocates of what we might call the far left and the far right. These two extremes can be described as the high carbohydrate vs. the low carbohydrate schools of thought. (You'll notice the ADA did not commit itself on the amount of carbohydrate allowed.) The most controversial aspect of diet has become the amount of carbohydrate allowed, because it is largely carbohydrate that accounts for the rise in blood sugar. (Carbohydrate foods are fruits, vegetables, milk, and all starches such as bread, rice, pasta, cereals, potatoes, and just about every dessert.) Dr. James Anderson of the Veterans Administration hospital in Lexington, Kentucky, has been a leader for the high carbohydrate diet, and Dr. Richard K. Bernstein is a principal advocate of the low carbohydrate diet.

Dr. James Anderson in his book of 1981, *Diabetes: A Practical New Guide to Healthy Living,* presents his High Carbohydrate/Fiber (HCF) nutrition plan which his studies show is particularly helpful for overweight, non-insulin-dependent diabetics. His diet formula is 55 to 60 percent carbohydrate, 12 to 20 percent protein, 20 to 25 percent fat, and 30 to 60 grams of fiber daily. The high fiber aspect of this diet is important because fiber slows down the absorption of sugars and starches in the intestine and helps keep your blood sugar from rising as high or as fast after a meal. This plan is very similar to a vegetarian diet.

Just the opposite diet is recommended by Dr. Richard K. Bernstein of Mamaroneck, New York. His book, *Dr. Bernstein's Diabetes Solution: A Complete Guide to Achieving Normal Blood Sugars,* emphasizes absolute normalization of blood sugar (a constant 90–95) by severely restricting carbohydrate to 6 grams at breakfast, 12 grams at lunch, and 12 grams at dinner. By way of example, one piece of one-ounce bread is 15 grams and one cup of milk is 12 grams, whereas meats, fish, and fats are largely carbohydrate-free. Dr. Bernstein's plan is perforce a high-protein-and-fat diet. He believes that "loading with carbohydrate will probably be more harmful in the long run than loading with fat." Dr. Bernstein, himself a diabetic for 50 years with no complications, is one physician who did heal himself! Since this is the most controversial of the diets and in some ways the most difficult to follow, we call his regime the "Dietary Court of Last Resort." A supplement at the end of this book gives you a detailed description of this diet, as well as a report of our own experience with it.

Which is the best dietary choice for me?

This question, of course, is the crux of the matter. You may need to use the try-and-see approach if the plan you're using is inadequate for blood-sugar control or unpleasing to the palate or both. One strict warning: If you are now using medication (pills or insulin), it is unsafe to change what you eat without the guidance of your doctor or health care team. At this point we want to prioritize for you the goals of diabetes dietary therapy so that you'll have a good perspective on this crucial, often confusing subject. The best diet for you is:

1. *The diet that best allows you to keep your blood sugar as close to normal as possible.* Only your blood-sugar tests can tell you if your diet is working. Another way to judge is by your A_1C test. How close to normal is it?

2. *The diet that keeps you healthy.* Important as it is to keep your diabetes under control, that's not enough. You're a whole living person, not just a pancreas, and you need to eat a healthy diet for that whole living person. We're always amused to see those exchange lists put out by fast-food establishments that make it look as if you could follow the exchanges, eat fast food for every meal of every day, and live healthily ever after. You can't. You need to follow the general principles of dietary health, just as everyone else interested in longevity and feeling good does.

3. *The diet that lets you enjoy your food.* Julia Child, the famous French-style gourmet cook, who's feisty and frisky at the age of eighty-five, complains that Americans are becoming afraid of food and are eating as if it were medicine, when they should be thinking of it as healthful and tasty and a pleasurable social experience. It is her opinion that "if we ate the way the nutritionists want us to, our teeth would be falling out, our hair would be falling out, and our skin would be drying up." On top of that we wouldn't be having any mealtime fun. Right on, Julia!

Since there are so many dietary considerations and options, we think that working with a dietitian is an excellent investment. And after July 1998 for those on Medicare it won't be such an investment, because Medicare will be covering dietary counseling for people with diabetes. It's best to seek out a registered dietitian (R.D.) who is also a

Certified Diabetes Educator (C.D.E.). For a referral, call the ADA's Division of Dietitians in Diabetes Care and Education: 1-800-877-1600, extension 4815, or the AADE: 1-800-338-3633.

There you have it. A smorgasbord of diabetes dining possibilities that you and your dietitian can select from to ensure your dining and blood-sugar happiness.

How can I make myself follow the diabetes diet?

You can conjure up horror stories in your imagination about the terrible things that will happen to you if you don't. But a strong, positive approach is better. Make your meals so delicious and interesting that you *want* to follow your diet. Make your eating not a grim therapy but a pleasurable delight. There are lots of gourmet cookbooks available for diabetics (see the reference section). Try new recipes. Try variations on old recipes. Try different herbs and spices (most of these are free, diabetically speaking). And don't overlook the aesthetics of food serving. A few flowers on the table give you no extra carbohydrates or calories and do a lot toward making mealtimes a pleasure.

This all holds especially true if you live alone. June, in her prediabetic days, often used to have for dinner what we called an "avocado sandwich maybe," since whenever someone asked her what she was having for dinner, she usually responded vaguely, "Oh, I guess I'll have an avocado sandwich maybe." Which meant she had no idea what she was going to have and didn't intend to make any plans. She was going to grab whatever she found in the refrigerator, if anything. Now June always has a well-planned and delicious meal served with style. In other words, she treats herself as an honored guest at her own table.

The most ghastly diabetic diet idea we've ever heard of is the result of one man's decision that calculating the diabetic diet is too much of a chore. He resolved to eat the same breakfast, the same lunch, and the same dinner every day. Ugh! Besides being lethally boring, this is nutritionally unsound. Diabetics need a lot of variety in their diets in order to make certain they're covering all the nutritional waterfronts. Not only that, but, as a home economist told us wryly, "you should eat a great variety of foods because there are so many chemicals in everything these days, it's the only way you can avoid getting a big buildup of one chemical that might cause harmful side effects."

Which foods are best for keeping my blood sugar normal?

First, as we pointed out before, it is mainly the carbohydrates in foods that are converted directly into glucose and affect your blood sugar. True, about 50 percent of protein becomes glucose, but since it takes six or eight hours to do so, it has more of a stabilizing than an escalating effect. Fat is not changed to glucose.

But all carbohydrates are not created equal. There was no scientific data on what effect individual carbohydrate foods have on blood sugar until 1983, when Dr. David Jenkins and fellow researchers at the University of Toronto published the Carbohydrate Glycemic Index. This is a classification of how high and how fast certain foods raise blood sugar. The problem with the index is that in compiling it only sixty-two foods were tested.

For diabetics, generally speaking, a food with a low (slow-releasing) glycemic index is preferred to one with a high (fast-releasing) index. The foods on the index are compared to glucose, which is assigned the top figure of 100. The findings are often surprising: sucrose (table sugar) is only 59, while carrots (cooked) are 92; instant potatoes are 80, but sweet potatoes are only 48. Ice cream is only 36, so index-wise it's as good for diabetics as lima beans, which are also 36. If you're thinking there must be a catch, there is. A bowl of ice cream has a lot more calories than a bowl of lima beans. In other words, you cannot and should not eat by glycemic index alone.

CARBOHYDRATE GLYCEMIC INDEX

SIMPLE SUGARS

Fructose—20

Sucrose—59

Honey—87

Glucose—100

FRUITS

Apples—39

Oranges—40

Orange Juice—46

Bananas—62

Raisins—64

STARCHY VEGETABLES

Sweet Potatoes—48

Yams—51

Beets—64

White Potatoes—70

Instant Potatoes—80

Carrots—92

Parsnips—97

DAIRY PRODUCTS

Skim Milk—32

Whole Milk—34

Ice Cream—36

Yogurt—36

LEGUMES

Soybeans—15

Lentils—29

Kidney Beans—29

Black-eyed Peas—33

Garbanzos—36

Lima Beans—36

Baked Beans—40

Frozen Peas—51

PASTA, CORN, RICE, BREAD

Whole-wheat Pasta—42

White Pasta—50

Sweet Corn—59

Brown Rice—66

White Bread—69

Whole-wheat Bread—72

White Rice—72

BREAKFAST CEREALS

Oatmeal—49

All-Bran—51

Swiss Muesli—66

Shredded Wheat—67

Cornflakes—80

MISCELLANEOUS

Peanuts—13

Sausages—28

Fish Sticks—38

Tomato Soup—38

Sponge Cake—46

Potato Chips—51

Mars Bars—68

It's also known that when carbohydrates are eaten as part of a meal that includes protein and fat rather than alone, blood sugar rises less. A further complication is that not all people respond to different kinds of carbohydrate in the same way. In a sense, you need to use your blood-sugar tests to figure out how you respond to different foods. You need to create your own glycemic index.

Though there are these drawbacks to the glycemic index, we find that it is for many people a very helpful guide to foods likely to help or hinder control. Eating more of the foods with an index of 50 or lower and less of those with higher ratings might make an encouraging difference to many of you who have been innocently consuming too many foods at the top of the scale.

For extensive information and updates on the glycemic index, check Rick Mendosa's glycemic index Web site: http:www.mendosa.com/gi.htm.

What is the carbohydrate counting that I'm starting to hear about?

Though the exchange system is an easy, basic, beginning way to design diabetic meals, of late a more precise system is being taught. Carbohydrate counting, as it's called, has you measure at each meal the exact amount (in grams, not ounces) of carbohydrate you intend to eat. The kind of carbohydrate is less important than the amount. This system has become increasingly popular because of the number of people now using intensive therapy (multiple shots of insulin daily or the insulin pump). Carbohydrate counting eliminates much of the guesswork of the past and gives a highly predictable result. It also simplifies insulin adjustment before meals.

The rationale for focusing solely on carbohydrates is that carbohydrate foods have a much greater impact on blood sugar than protein or fat. This means that the only portion of food that really needs to be covered by insulin (your own or injected) is the carbohydrate content of the food.

A first step is to decide how many grams of carbohydrate you want to eat at each meal or, preferably, how many grams your doctor or dietitian assigns you. This way your pre-meal insulin dose can be precisely calculated to cover that amount of carbohydrate. As an average, one unit of insulin will handle ten grams of carbohydrate, though this correspondence depends mostly on your type of diabetes and your individual response to insulin. Also adjustments are necessary depending on how high or low your blood sugar is before eating. (Nothing's as simple as we'd all like it to be!)

How do I find out how many grams of carbohydrate are in the food portions I'm going to eat?

It takes a bit of learning, but there are now many good sources of information. The two main reference tools are:

1. *The "Nutrition Facts" food labels on products you buy in the market.* These list the serving size and the total grams of carbohydrate in that size serving. You're probably acquainted with these already.

2. *Food composition books.* There are many available now, even in pocket size, such as the *Carbohydrate Addict's Gram Counter.* (See the reference section for several choices.) These tell you the number of grams of carbohydrate in a particular serving size. For instance, one cup of raw, unpeeled apple slices has 16.8 grams of carbohydrate; one Pepperidge Farms plain hamburger bun has 22 grams; a Celeste Suprema Pizza for One has 54 grams.

3. *A scale that weighs in grams* (we use the Swiss-made Soehnle Attaché) *and a booklet that lists the percentage of carbohydrate in foods.* A good one of these is *The Pocket Pancreas.* (See the reference section.) Weigh what you intend to eat, then look up the percentage of carbohydrate in that food. Using this method you find, for example, that an apple is 13 percent carbohydrate. If your apple (or piece of apple) weighs 60 grams, taking 13 percent of that tells you that it contains only 7.8 grams of carbohydrate. If you had half a bagel that weighed 70 grams (a little over 2 ounces), you would be eating 33.6 grams of carbohydrate, because a bagel is 56 percent carbohydrate.

An easier, albeit more expensive, way to go is to use the Soehnle computerized scale, the Diet/Health computer, with a databank of 380 foods. This scale automatically calculates the amount of carbohydrate plus other nutritional values in any food you weigh on it. It can even keep track of everything you eat and give you a readout at the end of the day.

Dietitian Betty Brackenridge has created an excellent, easy-to-understand audio cassette, *Carbohydrate Counting.* (See the reference section.)

Carbohydrate counting can help type 2's as well as type 1's to fine-tune their blood-sugar levels after meals. For everyone it is definitely a skill well worth learning.

If you're really conscientious at first about weighing and measuring your food, you'll be amazed at how quickly you learn to eye-measure or, as with bread, hand-weigh when you're out to dinner at a friend's house or in a restaurant. (Hint: sometimes it helps to discreetly nudge your food into little piles, the better to estimate the quantity.) You may get so good at eye-measuring and hand-weighing that you can do weight- and quantity-guessing parlor tricks, like the guy who guesses weights at the circus. Of course, the real and worthwhile trick is using your skill to eat the exact amount of food on your diet.

Can I have a light breakfast and lunch and a big dinner?

That's not a good idea for people with diabetes, especially when that big meal is at night. Your metabolism is slower at night and caloric needs lower than at any time during the day. Smaller, more frequent meals and snacks are the preferred way of life.

You'll get into real trouble by trying to follow the great American eating pattern of nothing much for breakfast, a light lunch, and a gorging session at night. According to the book *Outsmarting the Female Fat Cell,* by Debra Waterhouse, M.P.H., R.D., typical Americans eat 70 percent of their calories after five o' clock at night, whereas Europeans and other cultures eat their largest meal at midday. Her theory is that that's why these cultures do not have the weight problems that Americans do.

Studies have actually shown that type 1's who skip meals and eat one large meal at night have poor glucose tolerance, higher cholesterol levels, and, again, a tendency to be overweight. Type 2's run the same risks plus an even greater tendency for weight gain.

Is there anything I can eat all I want of without counting it in my diet?

You can hype up the flavors of your meals with herbs and spices without counting them. And you can eat as much of certain vegetables as you want, if you eat them raw: chicory; Chinese cabbage; endive; escarole; iceberg, butter, red-leaf, or romaine lettuce; parsley; watercress, and the like. There is a list of such "free foods" in *Exchange Lists for Meal Planning*.

Can I follow a vegetarian diet?

Yes, in fact many consider the vegetarian diet extremely healthy for everyone and especially good for non-insulin-dependent diabetics who are overweight. In fact, Dr. James Anderson's HCF diet (see reference to this diet on pages 41–42) is as close as it can get to a vegetarian diet without being one.

One advantage of vegetarianism is that the diet is naturally low in fat and high in fiber. Many of the staples of the diet—soybeans, beans, oats, lentils, pasta, brown rice—are low on the Carbohydrate Glycemic Index (see pages 46–47). This, along with their high fiber content, means that food becomes glucose at a slow pace and blood sugar stays normal more easily. In addition to helping control diabetes, a vegetarian diet reduces the risk of heart disease and tends to promote weight loss.

There is more than one type of vegetarian diet: *vegan,* or no animal food at all; *lacto-vegetarian,* all vegetable except for milk, cheese, and other dairy products; and *lacto-ovo-vegetarian,* in which both dairy products and eggs can be eaten. The problem with vegan is that calcium and iron may be in low supply, and a pill supplement may be advisable. The main problem with all vegetarian diets is that they can be deficient in vitamin B-12, which can be taken in pill form but is more effective when injected. So if you're an insulin taker and familiar with the injection process, you might ask your doctor about shooting your own B-12.

To follow a vegetarian diet as a diabetic, you need special food lists for guidance in calorie content and carbohydrate and fat amounts. The most complete lists we know of are in Marion Franz's *Exchanges for All Occasions*. Our favorite vegetarian cookbook is *The New Laurel's Kitchen*, by Laurel Robertson et al. which, unlike many such cookbooks, is not laden with sweets and fats. (See the reference section for a complete list of exchange lists and cookbooks.)

Will I be able to follow my diet in restaurants?

Of course. It won't be as easy as following it at home, where you can select and measure everything to make sure you're getting exactly what you need, but with a little experience and ingenuity it can be done. In fact, it is done by diabetics every day.

At first, when you're just getting started with diabetes, you might want to check out the restaurant ahead of time to see what they have on the menu that would be right for you. (If you have access to a fax machine, you can have the restaurant fax you a copy of its menu.) This gives you time to figure out in advance what you want to order. You can also find out if they have, for example, fruit for dessert rather than something gloppy and sweet.

Checking out the restaurant ahead of time is also a good idea because you'll know if it's open. Sometimes on a trip June has gone out to a restaurant recommended in a travel book or article only to find it's been closed for six months. This can be more than an awkward situation if it's time to eat and there's no other restaurant around.

For insulin-dependent diabetics, a reservation is very important. Even then, there can be a delay. That's why, if you take insulin, it's a good idea not to take your shot until you arrive at the restaurant and see if there is a wait. If you're using Humalog, Eli Lilly's ultra-fast-acting insulin, the problem is easily resolved, because you can inject your insulin just before ordering or even as the appetizer arrives.

What kinds of things should I order in restaurants?

As long as you avoid concentrated sweets, you can usually order any-thing you want. At first, though, try to avoid unfamiliar concoctions that are likely to have a lot of sauce (sauces often contain a great deal of car-bohydrate and fat). Straightforward poultry or fish, and bread and veg-etables, are the easiest things to recognize and measure.

This doesn't mean you're stuck with plain fare. There are several nutritional guides to help you make sound choices. You can select from *Exchanges for All Occasions* and *Fast Food Facts,* both by Marion Franz, R.D., or *The Restaurant Companion* by Hope S. Warshaw, R.D. (See the reference section.)

What do you mean by "concentrated sweets"?

Concentrated sweets are what, when you taste them, are sweet, all sweet, and nothing but sweet. They're sugar, honey, and syrup. They're candy, frosted cake, pies, cookies, and ice-cream sundaes. They're al-most everything listed on restaurant menus as desserts. They're all soft drinks, except artificially sweetened ones.

Concentrated sweets are an assault upon your system that sends your blood sugar soaring. Besides that, they quickly use up your daily allotment of calories without giving you any real food value in return—empty calories, as they're known.

Are there any sweeteners I can safely use?

Sweets are a problem for all of us. We seem to be biologically pro-grammed to like them. Our ancestors had to have this craving for sweets to inspire them to climb trees for fruit to get the vitamins they needed. Or it may be psychological, because we were rewarded with sweet treats when we were good little girls and boys, and we still seek that feeling of being loved and approved. Or it may be a combination of the two, and that makes it even harder to kick the sweets habit.

Let's talk first about the ubiquitous sugar (sucrose) before we take up the rest. You've probably been terrorized about even so much as looking at a grain of it. But now we're being told that a little bit of sugar is no problem in a well-balanced diet. Scientists have concluded that it does not cause a more rapid rise in blood-glucose levels than starch. Just don't eat more than 10 percent of your total carbohydrate calories in the form of sugar (they're empty calories) and never use it straight in drinks. As our type 2 book collaborator, Virginia Valentine, says, "You can have goodies such as low-sugar cookies (animal crackers, gingersnaps, vanilla wafers, etc.), low-sugar cakes with no icing, or low-sugar frozen yoghurt or ice cream."

There are two kinds of sweeteners: noncaloric and caloric. The noncaloric sweeteners include saccharine, aspartame (NutraSweet and Equal), DiabetiSweet, and Sunette (Sweet One). The most commonly used caloric ones besides sugar are fructose, sorbitol, mannitol, and HSH. Caloric sweeteners should not be "ingested freely," as dietitians like to put it. We actually don't feel that *any* sweetener should be ingested freely, since you never know when a laboratory mouse is going to clutch his bladder or liver and topple over and cause hysterical headlines about a previously approved sweetener. So again you have that good old boring admonition to practice moderation.

One way of achieving moderation is not to concentrate on one kind of sweetener but to vary them, never having more than a couple of items sweetened with any one kind of artificial sweetener a day. That way if the mouse topples, you won't have to worry that your system is loaded with lethals.

Following is a rundown of the various sweeteners and how to fit them into your diet.

Caloric Sweeteners

Fructose. There are several good things to say about fructose. First off, it's not an artificial sweetener. It is, as they like to say about almost every product you see in markets these days, "all natural." It is found in sweet fruit and most vegetables. It is also available in granular and liquid form in diabetes supply centers. It tastes sweet and has about the same calorie count as sugar (100 calories per ounce). But because it is much sweeter than sugar, you can use less of it to get the same sweet taste. The graph reprinted from *Laurel's Kitchen* shows how much sweeter it is.

Fructose also doesn't raise your blood sugar as fast or as high as sucrose. The Carbohydrate Glycemic Index (see pages 46–47) gives it a 20 as compared with a 59 for sucrose and a 100 for glucose. One caution: *If your blood sugar is already high, fructose will raise your blood sugar just as fast and as high as sugar.*

If you want to use fructose in baking, former dietitian (and now doctor) Ron Brown suggests that you use it for one-quarter of the sugar in the recipe and a noncaloric sweetener for another quarter. You can usually just leave out the rest, he says, since most desserts are too sweet anyway.

The British Diabetic Association reports that when you use fructose in cakes, it tends to keep them fresher longer and also has a better taste than ordinary sugar. The association does caution, however, in capital letters and boldface type: **FRUIT SUGAR IS NOT SUITABLE FOR THE OVERWEIGHT.**

There have been reports that fructose raises triglycerides (fats stored in the blood). However, at the 1993 ADA Scientific Sessions this fear was put to rest by John P. Bantle, M.D., with the statement that fructose has no effect on triglycerides. But it does raise cholesterol, primarily the LDLs (bad ones). This is now the main objection to fructose in the diabetic diet. Once again, moderation is the answer in using any kind of sweetener.

**RELATIVE SWEETNESS
OF SUGARS**
*Expressed as percentages of
sucrose or table sugar*

Fructose   173

Sucrose   100

Glucose   74

Maltose &
Galactose   33

Lactose   16

Reprinted by permission from Laurel's Kitchen by Laurel Robertson, Carol Flinders, and
Bronwen Godfrey (Nilgiri Press, 1976).

The terms *fructose* and *fruit sugar* are used interchangeably. In
England and Europe, fructose is usually made from fruit; in the United
States, it is made from corn. Fructose and fruit sugar are chemically the same, although some people claim there is a difference in
taste.

Sorbitol. Sorbitol, a sugar alcohol found in many plants, like fructose, doesn't cause the blood sugar to rise as rapidly as sugar because
of the way it's metabolized. Sorbitol suffers a bad press for its tendency
to have a laxative effect in certain susceptible people. (We think of that

as nature's way of promoting moderation.) We've also heard people denigrate sorbitol as an artificial sweetener. Not true. Sorbitol is found naturally in fruit. It was our friend Daisy Kuhn, professor of microbiology at California State University at Northridge, who put us straight on this. She even gave June a basket of prunes and pears as a sorbitol Easter gift, explaining that these two fruits are among the highest in sorbitol. This, of course, explains why prunes work so well as a laxative. Other fruits with a high sorbitol content are plums, berries, apples, and cherries. Daisy tells us that it is safe for most adults to eat about 40 grams of sorbitol if it is spaced out over a day. A three-ounce serving of prunes has about 12 grams of sorbitol. Hard candies sweetened with sorbitol contain about 2.6 grams. Though many commercial foods are sweetened with sorbitol, consumers in the United States cannot buy it for home use.

Another erroneous bum rap for sorbitol is that it causes the diabetes complications of retinopathy and neuropathy. This is a confusion between two different sorbitols. The sorbitol that does the damage is a waste product produced from glucose in the bloodstream. It is definitely *not* the sorbitol eaten as food. (Incidentally, an enzyme called aldose reductase stimulates the conversion of blood glucose into sorbitol. For that reason a new drug is being developed to block the action of aldose reductase and thereby to prevent the development of these diabetes complications.) To reiterate: *Sorbitol eaten as a food is not implicated in eye, nerve, or kidney damage.*

Mannitol. Mannitol, another sugar alcohol, is similar to sorbitol—including its laxitivity in susceptible individuals. It's also used as a commercial sweetening agent, although not as commonly as sorbitol.

HSH (Hydrogenated Starch Hydrolysate). Daisy Kuhn tells us that HSH is *chemically* the same as sorbitol. We've heard that it isn't quite as laxative as sorbitol, but since we've heard this mainly from companies that manufacture products made with HSH, we're waiting for more evidence to substantiate this claim. HSH is the sweetener in many sugar-free candies.

Noncaloric Sweeteners

People have very strong feelings about artificial sweeteners. Some won't touch them with a twelve-foot tongue. One woman called us in a fury to cancel her subscription to our newsletter because we mentioned Equal in it. And we once heard a lecture by a doctor, a medical adviser for an ADA chapter, in which he cited the many evils of saccharine, saying that it, and not cyclamates, should have been banned by the FDA. By the way, any of the artificial sweeteners tasted alone will taste anywhere from bad to funny. They taste good only in foods and drinks. Here, then, is a brief rundown of the current crop of artificial sweeteners.

Saccharine. This is the primary sweetening component of Sweet 'N Low and Sugar Twin. It can be used in cooking. Some people find that it has a bitter or metallic aftertaste, but when combined with fructose in a recipe it's not noticeable. Because saccharine has been known to cause cancer when fed to animals in huge amounts, the FDA requires all products containing saccharine to bear the following warning: "Use of this product may be hazardous to your health. This product contains saccharine, which has been determined to cause cancer in laboratory animals." Those studies haven't yet been directly correlated to humans.

Aspartame (NutraSweet and Equal). This is currently the most popular noncaloric sweetener around—and it is around everywhere. It doesn't have the aftertaste of saccharine, but its tragic flaw is that it loses its sweetness in cooking or baking and doesn't have enough bulk for baked goods. One packet of Equal is equivalent in sweetness to two teaspoons of sugar. One tablet equals one teaspoon of sugar.

Since aspartame can be harmful to people with a rare metabolic abnormality called PKU (phenylketonuria), the FDA requires that it carry a warning on the package. The FDA considers that an acceptable amount of aspartame is up to 50 milligrams per kilogram (2.2 pounds) of body weight. Gloria Loring, in her *Kids, Food, and Diabetes,* translates this as one twelve-ounce can of aspartame-sweetened soda per 12 pounds of body weight. Actually, a 132-pound person would have to consume eighty-six packets a day to reach the FDA's maximum accepted intake.

DiabetiSweet. The newest sweetener on the market is versatile enough to be used in any way that sugar is. It even has a granular texture and tastes better than most of the noncaloric ones, possibly because it's a combination of three separate sweeteners: isomalt, acesulfame potassium, and aspartame. It comes in packets, each of which is as sweet as two teaspoons of sugar. A packet has one gram of carbohydrate.

Sunette (Sweet One). Sunette was safely used outside the United States for five years before it was approved here. It's the only dietetic sweetener that doesn't require a warning label. (Apparently so far nary a mouse has toppled.) Sunette is two hundred times sweeter than sugar. Its big advantage is that it doesn't break down when heated; therefore, you can cook with it. Each packet gives the sweetness of two teaspoons of sugar, and each contains four calories and one gram of carbohydrate. The carbohydrate is in the form of dextrose. "Not to worry," says dietitian Meg Gaekle. "It's added only to give bulk." (The manufacturers of Sweet 'N Low do the same thing.) In the small amounts generally used, it causes no problems.

A final reminder: Honey, molasses, pure maple syrup, and other such sweeteners are not approved for diabetics, no matter how many ill-informed health-food-store people tell you they are. (For more information on sweeteners, see "How Sweet It Is" in the reference section.)

What do I do if I am served too much food?

Leave what you can't eat or, in the case of expensive protein, take it home with you in a doggie bag. (You may have enough meat to last you for two or three meals.) June has the trick of carrying plastic bags in her purse and quietly bagging any excess.

One way to avoid getting plates that are bursting with calories is to go to restaurants that feature California or spa cuisine. But don't be sad if there aren't any of these in your area. They are usually very expensive, and you can actually sometimes get too little food in such establishments.

A happy trend in restaurant menus is the appearance of special "Pritikin Plates" and American Heart Association selections. These are low in calories and fat and high in fiber; watch for them. You should also watch for the restaurants that have special "light eater" dinners. There aren't many of these, but there are more and more all the time, because more and more people want to watch their weight or, as in the case of older people, just have diminished appetites.

Another way to get a smaller portion if you're dining with a cooperative person is to order one entree and split it. Each of you can then have an individual choice of appetizer. This limits both the amount of food and its price.

Our favorite trick for getting smaller portions and saving money and yet experiencing the best of dining out is to go for lunch rather than dinner. The portions are about half as large, with prices to match. A further advantage is that you're eating your main meal in the middle of the day, so you can walk it off afterward rather than just going to bed on a full stomach and letting it turn to fat. We especially do this main-meal-at-lunch trick when we travel. Dinner is then something light in the hotel coffee shop, or something we bring into the room.

Are salads always a safe bet when you're confused about what to order?

Let's take the ubiquitous salad bar, for example. It can be hazardous to your health in several ways. People sometimes cough and sneeze over salad bars, and to keep the ingredients fresh-looking, they are often sprayed with allergy-causing sulfides. But worst of all, while you think you're restricting yourself to a diet meal, you're actually loading up on calories from the dressing. One study showed that the average person takes in more calories from a salad bar than he or she would from a standard meat-and-potatoes lunch.

It's not always that much better if the salad is brought to your table. As *Better Homes and Gardens* reported, a chef's salad with cheese, ham, turkey, and half an egg dolloped with blue-cheese dressing has seven hundred calories and 58 grams of fat. For less than half the calories and 10 percent of the fat you can have a turkey sandwich made with two slices of whole-wheat bread, lettuce, and tomato.

Since dressing is the major culprit in a salad's assault on your diet, the only way to order salad is with dressing on the side. Then don't dump big globs onto your salad, but use this little trick a dieter once taught us: Dip your fork into the salad dressing and then pick up the lettuce or other vegetable with the fork. Just enough dressing clings to the fork and is transported to the salad to give it flavor with minimal calories.

How can I stay on my diet when I'm invited out to dinner?

First, make sure that anyone who invites you to dinner knows you're diabetic. That shouldn't be difficult, because people who know you well enough to extend the invitation will probably have long since been informed about your diabetes.

Almost anyone who knows you're diabetic will ask what's special about your diet. An easy way to explain it is to show the person the answer to the question "How do I plan a meal for my diabetic friend?" (see the section "For Family and Friends"). You might add that any vegetable is fine, except those root vegetables high on the Glycemic Index, such as cooked carrots, parsnips, and beets.

Another strategy was suggested by the Reverend Gerald Eaton, of Nicholasville, Kentucky. When he travels to other churches to preach, he sends an explanatory dietary sheet ahead to the host church. This is for those who will be providing him with meals. He just tells them he's on a "special diet" and not that he has diabetes, because if they have a diabetic "Aunt Susie" who doesn't watch her diet, he doesn't want them to think he can eat her way.

How do I make it through the holidays without breaking my diet?

Remember the origin of holiday festivals? They were the few occasions in the year when peasants who ran around most of the time with hollow, rumbling stomachs could really fill up. Now, however, most of the people in this country aren't perpetually hungry. On the contrary, what a biologist friend of ours calls "hyperalimentation," or eating too much, is a national epidemic. The American public's overeating habits are bad enough the whole year round, but then along come the holidays with the atavistic excuse for overindulgence, and the scene becomes a dietary disaster area.

Revelers sometimes rationalize their holiday behavior by quoting the philosopher who said, "What you eat and drink between Thanksgiving and New Year's isn't all that important. What really counts is what you eat and drink between New Year's and Thanksgiving." Of course, this philosopher didn't have diabetes. Diabetes doesn't take a holiday, and a diabetic can't take a holiday from health. So what are you to do?

Now, although there are gatherings where you won't be tempted by alcohol over the holidays (for the problem of avoiding alcohol, see "Can I drink alcohol?" on page 67), there's almost nowhere you can go where you won't be tempted by food, especially sugary food. With visions of sugarplums dancing in everyone's heads and on everyone's tables, it's going to take all your ingenuity to stick to your diet or, as we prefer to think of it, your healthful eating plan.

Let's take the last first—dessert. It's not uncommon to find two kinds of pie plus fruitcake, cookies, ice cream, whipped cream, and candy being offered with nary a morsel of plain fruit in sight. A gracious alternative is to bring your host or hostess a fruit-and-nut gift basket. You can call it a "diabetic dessert basket" and hope you'll be offered a chance to partake of it at the end of the meal.

Another way to avoid the dessert problem and yet still make the host or hostess happy is to take *one spoonful*. After all, if you've tasted the concoction, you can praise it, and that's the most important thing. It's also a way to make yourself feel less deprived.

Let's face the final reality, though. No matter how careful you are at a big holiday dinner, you're still likely to eat more than usual. But there is one survival tactic. Exercise more than usual. Do as much of the cooking and serving as you can arrange to. If you're going to someone else's house, tell the host or hostess in advance that you'd like to help pass things, clear the table, do anything that involves motion. Most people don't realize the physical effort that goes into serving a dinner. A few Thanksgivings ago June virtually singlehandedly put on a family holiday dinner, and although she ate a good bit more than her normal diet, that night she had the worst low-blood-sugar incident of her life.

After dinner is over keep the exercises going if you can. Organize a bird- or star-viewing walk, a caroling session, a tree-trimming activity, charades with lots of physical motion—anything to keep the calories burning and the blood sugar normal. The nicest part about all these activities is that they're enjoyable in themselves.

By the way, an after-dinner activity suggested by a former president of the ADA, Dr. Donald Bell, is testing the whole family's blood sugar. Since everyone will have had an abnormally heavy meal, it will be an appropriate time to see how their bodies handled it. Because there are those genetic factors to diabetes, you may catch a relative in the beginning stages, and he or she can get an early start on controlling it before any damage has been done. It may sound a little bizarre, but it's a good idea.

What happens if I break my diet?

If you do it once, you'll probably do it again and again and again. And each time you do it and run your blood sugar up, you risk damage to the body and the development of the serious complications of diabetes—heart disease and stroke, blindness, kidney and nerve damage, and gangrene of the feet.

The classic rationalizations are "Once won't hurt," "I can get away with it," "It's Christmas," "I can't offend the hostess," "It's my birthday," and "I'll be conspicuous if I don't." Consider yourself in a worse predicament than an alcoholic. He or she has to be a total abstainer from alcohol. You have to be a semi-abstainer from food, half on and half off the wagon at all times. A very precarious perch.

There are, however, three exceptions when we think it is okay to go ahead and break your diet. In fact, we heartily recommend it. These exceptions are: (1) the day you win a gold medal at the Olympics, (2) your inaugural banquet when you're elected President of the United States, and (3) your one-hundredth-birthday party.

Of course, after all this preaching, we admit that accidents will happen. Sometimes, for example, you'll inadvertently eat something that will be loaded with sugar. When you find yourself registering a high blood sugar after such an accident, there's no need for self-flagellation and heavy mourning. Occasional *accidental* lapses won't destroy you. (In fact, torturing yourself with frets and recriminations may do more damage to you than the dietary lapse.)

And, finally, to prove that we aren't as hard-line as we usually seem, we offer for your consideration the Hog Wild variation (see "For Family and Friends": "If my diabetic child goes to a birthday party or trick-or-treating on Halloween, is it all right to break the diet just this once?" on page 182). But at the same time, we want to warn you that wild hogs can easily get out of hand and break down all barriers of self-control, and to assure you that June does not practice the Hog Wild variation. *Ever.*

Is it all right to drink sugar-free and diet sodas?

These drinks are a great breakthrough for diabetics since they allow you to be part of the group without breaking your diet. As with all things, though, a bit of moderation is in order. We heard of one man who was downing over twenty cans of sugar-free soda a day. He must have sloshed when he walked, to say nothing of the excess chemicals that must have been assailing his system.

When it comes to sugar-free drinks, a bit of caution is also in order. True story: Once when June was skiing in Deer Valley, Utah, she felt very thirsty at the end of the day. The thing she wanted most was to try a glass of the locally brewed beer, Wasatch Gold. But she'd neglected to bring her testing things along to the slopes and felt she couldn't risk the carbohydrates. Therefore, like the conscientious diabetic that she is, June marched over to the soft-drink dispenser, filled a carton with sugar-free cola, and drank it all down.

When she got back to the lodge she tested her blood sugar. It was 220! She couldn't figure it out. She'd been exercising heavily all day and had eaten and drunk only the right things. Why the high blood sugar? Our conclusion was that it had to be the cola. The person who had filled the dispenser must have used the wrong cola mix, either mistakenly or because they were out of the sugar-free variety.

We thought this was an isolated occurrence until we were talking with the former president of the AADE, Kansas City diabetologist William Quick. He said that he and some patients and colleagues had conducted an experiment in fast-food chains in Kansas City and in Harrisburg, Pennsylvania. They tested the allegedly sugar-free drinks and discovered that one-third of them actually contained sugar.

You can test your own sugar-free drinks by carrying Tes-Tape or Diastix (for checking sugar in the urine); dip the strip or stick in the glass of soda and see how it registers.

As far as we know, soft drinks in cans are safe since their quality control is a little tighter than in mix-it-yourself establishments.

You also have to train family members and friends to watch what they're buying—and pouring. After twenty years of unmitigated alertness in sugar-free drink dispensing, Barbara absentmindedly bought a bottle of Schweppes tonic water that wasn't. For two evenings June drank it, wondering why her blood sugar was suddenly out of control every night. ("Am I coming down with something?") When she discovered the error, she was relieved to find that her diabetes hadn't become unpredictable. She was irritated with Barbara for her faulty purchase—but more irritated with herself for not taking the responsibility to always look for herself.

And a final warning on sugar-free sodas for type 1 diabetics: just when you get everyone thoroughly trained to give you sugar-free drinks and nothing but sugar-free drinks, you'll probably have an insulin reaction and ask for someone to bring you a Coke *quick* and they'll dutifully grab a sugar-free one, which will do about as much good for raising your blood sugar as a cup of air. (That's another reason for always using glucose tablets for hypoglycemia: they don't make sugar-free glucose tablets.)

Why am I supposed to read the label on all food products I buy? Aren't all brands more or less alike?

Brands are not only *not* alike, they are very different. Only by reading the fine print on the label can you know, for instance, whether a certain can of grapefruit juice contains sugar. Some brands do and some don't, and it's important for you to choose a brand that is unsweetened.

It's amazing how many food products have sugar thrown in. Fruits in heavy syrup are typical. You have to really search to find the few fruits, frozen or canned, that are unsweetened. Cans of vegetables often contain sugar, as do canned meats, bottled salad dressings, frozen dinners, and endless other convenience foods. Even *salt* contains sugar—read the label if you doubt us.

There's also a confusion about many diet products. You have to realize that the term *artificially sweetened* does not necessarily mean without sugar. Drinks sweetened with saccharine often contain some sugar to counteract saccharine's bitter taste. On low-cal foods, watch for the words *sugarless* and *sugar free*. But even that's not a guarantee of safety. By law only sucrose counts as sugar, so you'll have to watch for the many chemical terms used to specify different kinds of sugars: glucose, fructose, dextrose, maltose, lactose, dextrin, and sorbitol—just to name a few (see "How Sweet It Is" in the reference section for a complete list).

Incidentally, ingredient lists on labels are arranged according to the weight of each ingredient in descending order. The heaviest is listed first; the lightest, last. The lightest ingredients are usually those unintelligible chemical additives for which American food processors have become famous.

Can I drink alcohol?

Here you have one of the great diabetes controversies. Many doctors say absolutely no to alcohol. Not a drop. Others say it's all right in moderation. June has a joke that has a grain of truth in it. Question: "What did you do when your doctor said you couldn't drink?" Answer: "I changed doctors."

Actually, an excellent case can be made for a diabetic not to drink at all. Even alcoholic beverages that don't contain carbohydrate, such as gin, vodka, bourbon, scotch, and dry wines, do contain calories. If you have a weight problem, the additional calories of the drink will augment this problem. If you say, "Okay, I'll figure the calories of the drink in my diet and cut out something else," you will lose the food value of that something else you cut out and your body will be deprived of the nutrition it needs.

Then, too, drinking can get you in deep trouble, especially if you're on insulin. Alcohol lowers blood sugar unless you eat while you're drinking. If you start staggering or become unconscious on the way back to your car after a visit to a bar, the police will smell the alcohol and think you're simply drunk. This is not a scenario with a happy ending.

There is the additional possibility that the alcohol may throw off your medication or alter the effect of your insulin. Some oral drugs combined with alcohol can cause nausea, sweating, and dizziness. And an out-of-control diabetic shouldn't drink a drop.

Heavy drinking can result in long-range problems for a diabetic. The journal *Diabetes Care* reported a study by David McCullogh and others of over five hundred diabetic men. The heavy drinkers in the group had a much higher incidence of painful diabetic neuropathy than the others did.

The case *for* drinking is weaker than the one against it. For many people a glass of wine is a pleasurable adjunct to a meal. It is, in fact, for some national groups as much a part of the meal as the food. There is also the "French paradox" that people who drink two or three glasses a day of red wine (or white, according to a Kaiser Permanente Medical Center study) have a lower risk of coronary heart disease. Researchers do point out that wine drinkers may have other traits, such as a more healthy diet, that protect them. (But remember, *heavy* drinking *causes* heart disease.)

Even with your doctor's approval, however, before having a glass of anything you should do a little self-analysis of your drinking habits. We have a philosophy about diabetic drinking that we think holds true. There are two situations where a diabetic should *not* drink: The first is if alcohol means nothing to you, and the second is if alcohol means everything to you.

Whatever you drink has to be figured into your meal plan and the calories counted. Alcoholic drinks are usually calculated as fat exchanges, although you can also substitute them for bread exchanges. Naturally, you can't mix liquor with orange juice or tomato juice without counting those exchanges also. And you have to avoid such mixers as ginger ale, tonic, and other sweetened soft drinks.

The alcoholic drinks that don't contain sugar or carbohydrates are dry white wines (including champagne), dry red and rosé wines, white vermouth, whiskey, gin, vodka, scotch, rum, brandy, and tequila. A four-ounce glass of wine is about 80 calories; a four-ounce glass of vermouth is about 140 calories. The hard liquors are calculated according to their proof. The higher the proof, the more calories. As an example, eighty-six-proof alcohol is 71 calories an ounce; one hundred–proof alcohol is 83 calories an ounce. Beer is 156 calories per twelve-ounce bottle, but it also contains about the same amount of carbohydrates as a bread exchange (13 grams). Light beer is only 90 calories on the average and contains the equivalent of one-half a bread exchange in carbohydrate. Liqueurs and cordials have to be avoided entirely as they contain sugar—sometimes as much as 50 percent sugar. Appetizer and dessert wines, like sweet sherry, port, and muscatel, are also too sweet for diabetics.

The general recommendation is to limit alcoholic beverages to 6 percent of your daily caloric allotment. For instance, if you're on a 1,500-calorie-a-day diet, you could have one four-ounce glass of wine (80 calories) or one generous ounce of eighty-six–proof liquor (71 calories) in soda or a sugar-free mixer. You could also have it in orange juice, if you counted that as one of your fruit exchanges. If you are on a 3,000-calorie-a-day diet, you could drink twice that much (but you wouldn't *have* to, of course).

Another solution is to limit your drinking to the nonalcoholic wines and beers now available. Ariél Vineyards of California produces award-winning alcohol-free wines that have less than half the calories of wines with alcohol. Zuri of Germany has a nonalcoholic Rhine wine that contains only 130 calories per bottle. Many alcohol-free beers are now on the market in different parts of the country.

Is caffeine bad for a diabetic?

Denise Webb, Ph.D (nutrition), R.D., writing in *Parade* magazine, November 16, 1997, answers the question succinctly and definitively: "Coffee, the much maligned brew, has been accused of causing everything from cancer to infertility. But experts now generally agree that there is no consistent scientific evidence to prove coffee is detrimental to your health."

We've been following the conversion of coffee from bad guy to good guy in our *Diabetic Reader* for several years, because our enjoyment of this aromatic and satisfying beverage has always been tempered with a feeling of guilt. We've hated to see it maligned, because not only is it a safe mood elevator but also, diabetically speaking, it's free—it contains no calories, carbohydrates, or fat. The following data should restore your confidence and relieve you of your fears.

The chemicals in coffee (both caffeinated and decaffeinated) may form potent antioxidants, similar to vitamin C or vitamin E, which are believed to help prevent cancer. Dr. Takayuki Shibamoto, a professor of environmental toxicology at the University of California at Davis, has reported that his preliminary study indicates that "the antioxidants in a cup of coffee might be equal to the amount found in three oranges." The only rule is that you have to drink your coffee within about the first twenty minutes after it's brewed to benefit from the antioxidants. We'll drink to that and to Dr. Shibamoto! Starbucks, here we come.

DIABETES AND YOUR HEALTH

What should I expect from my doctor?

Maybe we should start off with a modification of the question: "What should I expect from my doctor when first diagnosed?" This is a crucial time for you. We hope you received the examination, treatment, and care you needed and deserved at that time.

In order to give you an idea of what a first visit should involve, we consulted endocrinologist Dr. Michael Bush, director of the Diabetes Outpatient Training and Education Center at the Cedars-Sinai Medical Center in Los Angeles. He supplied a detailed account of what an ideal physical examination should be. (See "Doctor's Initial Examination" in the reference section.)

After your first visit, you'll need to follow your doctor's recommendations for how often he or she wants to see you. It might be as frequently as three or four times a month at first. Once you get over your initial learning period and the doctor feels you're ready to be more independent, your visits may be cut down to once every three months, especially if he or she wants to order laboratory tests, such as a hemo-globin A_1C test. At each visit the doctor needs to check your testing records and go over your self-care with you to see where improvements and changes should be made. This is also your chance to ask any questions you've come up with since your last office visit.

Your doctor should also be available by telephone (or have a colleague who is available) at all times in case any serious diabetes-related emergency develops and you need help. The doctor should be willing to answer occasional questions by phone when you're having trouble handling some diabetes problem.

All this is just standard care, however. The more important expectations you should have deal with your doctor's attitudes and your interaction with him or her.

First and foremost, you should expect your doctor to treat you as an individual, not just a textbook diabetes case. You are a person with definite needs and interests and likes and dislikes, and they can and should be incorporated into your treatment. There are many different ways of handling diabetes—different diets, different exercise plans, different pills, different insulin-injection schedules that can make diabetes come at least halfway toward adjusting to your life-style.

In order for the doctor to make these variations on the basic theme of diabetes care, she or he is going to have to spend a little time finding out about you and your way of living, working, and playing. In other words, your doctor is going to have to talk to you. No, make that talk *with* you. There should be an interchange of ideas, not a lecture. The doctor should regard you as a colleague in your diabetes care and never convey the idea that you are incapable of understanding your condition and treatment. In fact, as Dr. Donnell B. Etzwiler says: "Diabetic patients provide 99 percent of their own care." So as your own physician you'd *better* be capable of understanding your condition and its treatment.

Your doctor, therefore, should give you a full explanation of all the laboratory tests you have. Rather than telling you your blood sugar is "normal" or "a little high, but still okay," he or she should tell you the exact figures. You should also know exactly where you stand with cholesterol, triglycerides, blood pressure—everything that affects your health and that you can make better or worse by your own behavior.

Now, although there are a lot of things that your doctor has to discuss with you, we don't want to lead you to expect that the doctor should have long, leisurely conversations with you, going over every facet of your physiological and psychological makeup. A doctor's time is too valuable to squander in great chunks. You are not the only patient, and others have their needs, too.

And speaking of time, *your* time has some value, too. You deserve a doctor who doesn't overbook and keep patients crouching in the waiting room for hours, building up stresses that are very bad for diabetes control.

This is not to say you should *never* have to wait. There are emergencies that a doctor must handle, and they can throw the schedule off, but if there is an emergency every time you have an appointment, you have cause for suspicion. We wouldn't carry on about waiting time to this extent except that since most diabetics go to the doctor regularly every two or three months *forever,* that waiting-room time can really add up.

Since most doctors frankly admit that they lack a background in nutrition—one doctor told us he had had only a one-hour lecture on it during his entire time at medical school—you should expect your doctor to be able to refer you to a good dietitian to help you plan the complexities and personal variations of your diet. He or she shouldn't just throw a one-page diet list at you and send you on your way, or tell you that old myth, "Just don't eat sugar."

It is also extremely helpful if the office has a diabetes nurse specialist (a C.D.E.) (see page 44) who can help you develop a good technique with injections, blood-sugar testing, diet, and problems of daily living. Again, these are specifics that the doctor doesn't have the time to help you with.

You should expect your doctor to keep up with the latest developments in the field of diabetes and be willing to incorporate them into your treatment.

Finally—and this may be asking too much—we personally feel that your doctor and other involved health professionals should also provide a good example. It's rather difficult for you to take good health advice from a flabby chain-smoker who is obviously ignoring all such counsel.

From all these "shoulds," you can see that it helps a great deal if your doctor is a diabetologist or an internist who specializes in diabetes. Of course, if you are a member of an HMO, your medical care may be relegated to a family practitioner, and it's not always easy to get referred to a specialist in diabetes. Is this necessarily a drawback? Let us quote from a letter we received from Leslie Hayes, M.D., of the Health Centers of Northern New Mexico after we published an article in our *Diabetic Reader* about the difficulties of getting to see a specialist in HMOs:

> While I appreciate the frustration that your readers may feel about the HMO system, I would disagree that all diabetics need to see a specialist for regular medical care. More important than the type of specialist is the doctor herself. Finding a doctor who keeps herself well-educated, knows her limitations and whom you feel you can trust is essential. If you can find this doctor, then regardless of whether this person is a family practitioner, internist, or specialist, I would urge you to do anything you can to convince your HMO that she is whom you need to see.

How do I find a doctor who specializes in diabetes?

Doctors specializing in diabetes are usually listed under endocrinology and metabolism in the Yellow Pages. But rather than just sticking a pin in the telephone directory, you may prefer to call your local diabetes association and ask for the names of diabetologists who are closest to your home (and closeness *is* important). If your town has no local association, call your state affiliate of the ADA and ask for a recommendation.

If you still have no luck, call your local hospital and ask who on its staff handles most of the diabetes cases.

Another good thing to do is go to your public library and check the *Directory of Medical Specialists.* This way you can find out the doctor's training, what hospitals he or she has worked in, age, and special experience. (This book is a little tricky to use. You may need to ask the librarian for help.)

We realize, however, that in some small towns there simply isn't a diabetologist. In that case, find (or keep) a doctor with whom you feel you can have a good relationship. Look for one who is willing to explore solutions to problems you present. Be sure she or he is willing to investigate new developments in diabetes that you may learn about in your reading or from discussions at meetings and seminars.

Incidentally, if you have a beloved family doctor, there's no reason to desert him or her for a diabetologist. You can keep the beloved one as your general physician and go to your diabetologist for special diabetes care.

When your diabetes is in its early stages or if you start developing problems at any time, you may want to go to one of the major diabetes clinics in the country where you stay a week or so and are given examinations and lab tests. You attend classes and learn what you need to do to get your diabetes under good control.

After all this talk about what your doctor should do for you, we mustn't forget your responsibilities to your doctor and what your doctor should expect from you.

What should my doctor expect from me?

Number one is honesty. Always tell the doctor the truth about what you're doing (or not doing) in your diabetes care. Report the true results of your blood-sugar tests. (One young woman told us she faked the results of the tests because she didn't want the doctor to be disappointed.) The doctor can't get you on the right track if he or she doesn't know that you're on the wrong one. Never try to fake the doctor out by behaving like a model diabetic for the few days just before you're scheduled for an examination and being very casual (sloppy) about your self-care the rest of the time.

You also owe your doctor cooperation. If you can't or won't follow the advice you're given, you should find another doctor whose advice you can and will accept.

Your doctor should also be able to expect you to take good care of yourself—not just your diabetes, but your *whole self.* Too many of us think we can neglect our health or even actively destroy it and then go to the doctor and say, "I'm sick. Make me well." Then if the doctor can't rectify the damage we've done, we get angry.

Don't take advantage of your doctor. If you phone constantly to discuss every little problem or try to monopolize his or her time in the office, using the doctor as a father or mother confessor, you're actually taking advantage of other patients whose time you're usurping.

It's ironic, but once you've found a doctor who is willing to listen, you have to be responsible enough to restrain yourself and stick to the facts of your diabetes problem. True, your personal problems *are* a part of the total picture of your diabetes, but a mention of their existence is enough. A diabetologist is not a psychiatrist and cannot be expected to straighten out your marriage, assuage your guilt feelings, release your inhibitions, or do whatever else is required to give you psychic peace.

If your life problems weigh unbearably upon you and you feel they are significantly detrimental to your diabetes control, ask your doctor to recommend a therapist to help you with them.

How much should I weigh?

A better question would be "What percentage of my body weight should be fat?" The old height-weight-age tables are no longer considered good guides. Rather, correctness of weight should be determined by measuring the proportion of body fat and lean tissue. Simply weighing your-self is deceptive because muscle weighs more than fat, and it's the pro-portion of muscle to fat that counts from a health standpoint. In fact, you can be thin and still carry more fat than is healthy. When we spon-sored a health-fair day at the Sugar-Free Center in Van Nuys, our thinnest employee—you can almost see through her—turned out to be too fat, and she was advised to lose some fat and build up more muscle.

The recommended proportion of body fat is different for men and women. Men should be between 6 and 23 percent fat and women be-tween 9 and 30 percent, depending on age. Men who are 25 percent fat and women who are 35 percent fat are classified as obese. There is some controversy about these recommended figures, because this is a new concept, but since you already have diabetes as a risk factor it would seem wisest to play it safe and go for the lower end of the scale if at all possible (see table on next page).

In the first edition of this book we recommended a simple pinch test to see if you were too fat. You pinch up your flesh just below your ribs at your waistline. Pressing the flesh between your thumb and fore-finger, you should find a thickness of between one-half and one inch. If the pinch test reveals more flesh than that, you're too fat.

A more precise way, one that will predict the exact percentage of fat, is a caliper test. This is done by taking pinches with a caliper at the midriff, on the chest, just below the shoulder, and on the front of the thigh. These results are averaged, and a table gives the corresponding fat percentage. The caliper test must be taken in a doctor's office or at a fitness center.

The most accurate body-composition test is naturally the most awkward and expensive. For this, you need to be weighed underwater using a hydrodensitometer. Since fat floats and muscle sinks, the heav-ier you are underwater, the better. (It's the opposite of the situation on land.)

It seems to us that every diabetic should seek out a place to have one of these tests and find out his or her body composition. The tests are generally available at university medical centers, weight-loss clin-

RECOMMENDED PERCENT BODY FAT

AGE GROUP

Males	19–24	25–29	30–34	35–39	40–44	45–49	50–59	60+
Minimum (%)	6	6	6	6	6	6	6	6
Maximum (%)	14.8	16.5	18.0	19.4	20.5	21.5	22.7	23.5
Females								
Minimum (%)	9	9	9	9	9	9	9	9
Maximum (%)	21.9	22.4	22.7	23.7	25.4	27.2	30.0	30.8

Although there is no established "standard" for recommended percent body fat, this table is based on the consensus of many experts in the health field. (Copyright 1987, Futrex, Inc. Reprinted by permission.)

ics, health clubs, fitness centers, and some doctors' offices and sports-medicine centers. Incidentally, if you are overweight according to weight charts you could find out the happy news that your weightiness is mostly due to muscle and therefore not risky at all. In fact, researchers did a study that proved that overweight lean men have the same low risk of developing heart disease as normal-weight lean men. Only overweight fat men are at greater risk.

Do I have to worry about cholesterol?

Everyone these days is either worrying about cholesterol or worrying about whether they should be worrying about it. Still cholesterol is something you should take seriously, especially if you have diabetes. Diabetics are more likely to have higher levels of cholesterol and blood fats (triglycerides). It may be that high blood sugar causes elevation of LDLs (low-density lipoproteins, or "bad" cholesterol) and lowering of HDLs (high-density lipoproteins, or "good" cholesterol). HDLs are thought to remove cholesterol from the arteries, while LDLs lead to fatty deposits that clog the arteries and cause heart attacks.

What should your cholesterol level be? The old consensus was that it should be under 200 milligrams of cholesterol per deciliter of blood; 240 was considered borderline high risk. Nowadays heart risk is not judged by your total cholesterol so much as by the ratio between the good HDLs and the bad LDLs. You can actually have fairly high total cholesterol and still be without heart risk if your HDLs are high enough. The recommended level of HDL is over 50 and of LDL is 130 or less.

According to Drs. Michael and Mary Dan Eades, in their book *Protein Power,* the way to calculate your heart risk is to divide your total cholesterol by your total HDL. The result should be below four. Then divide you LDL by your HDL; this result should be below three.

It stands to reason that all diabetics should have regular cholesterol tests to make sure they're keeping their risk level low enough. Diet and exercise can improve cholesterol levels. Oat bran can help reduce cholesterol; in fact, the FDA has approved allowing it to be labeled as cholesterol-lowering. Eggs have always been considered taboo in every health-conscious person's diet because each yolk has 315 milligrams of cholesterol, which is more than the 300 milligrams we should limit ourselves to each day. Lately, however, Humpty Dumpty is starting to get put together again. Eggs have made somewhat of a comeback. Several comprehensive studies suggest that moderate eating of eggs may pose no problem for generally healthy adults. It seems that only people with a combination of high blood cholesterol and triglycerides need to cut back on eggs. Most researchers believe now that saturated fats in the diet are more likely to raise blood cholesterol levels than dietary cholesterol.

Do I have to exercise?

A better question would be "Isn't it terrific that such an enjoyable activity as exercise is a basic part of diabetes therapy?" The answer to both questions is yes.

Although exercise is often a neglected area in diabetes care, getting the right amount of exercise is just as important as following a good eating plan—if not more important.

We've heard it said that if you had to make a choice between eating junk food and exercising or eating a perfectly healthy diet and being immobile, you'd be healthier eating the junk food and exercising. Of course, you don't have to make that choice—in fact, you can't make it. You need both exercise and good food for optimum health and blood-sugar control.

Exercise is almost a magic formula for diabetics. If you're too thin—usually the lean, insulin-dependent types—it will help you gain needed pounds by causing you to utilize your food better. Since it acts like an "invisible insulin," it helps get glucose into the cells, so less is wasted by being spilled into the urine.

If you're overweight, exercise will help you lose weight—and keep it off. Contrary to the myth, exercise does *not* increase your appetite. In fact, it suppresses it by regulating your *appestat,* the brain center that controls the appetite, and redirecting the blood flow away from the digestive tract. As a result, you'll be able to eat more because of the calories you burn, yet you'll feel like eating less. This combination will deliver you from that complaint of so many diabetics: "I'm always hungry."

Exercise also makes weight loss easier because it revs up your metabolism, with the result that you burn more calories even when you're sitting still or sleeping. This principle is explained in Covert Bailey's well-known book *The New Fit or Fat?*

Besides helping overweight type 2 diabetics lose weight, exercise lowers blood sugar by actually increasing the number of insulin receptors—those cell "locks" into which the key of insulin is inserted.

Exercise helps all of you improve circulation and lower blood fats (cholesterol and triglycerides) and therefore helps ward off the heart and blood-vessel problems to which diabetics are subject.

The benefits of exercise are not limited to physical improvements. Exercise lessens stress and is a great mood elevator. Perhaps you've heard of those brain chemicals called endorphins. Endorphins are known as the morphine within and are released when you exercise. They give you a natural high such as runners experience after about a half hour. This kind of morphine is a drug worth getting hooked on.

The only tragedy associated with exercise is that of people who have physical problems that prevent them from doing it. Those of you who have proliferative retinopathy are warned that exercise may aggravate the problem. People with heart disease should also be aware of exercise cautions and check with their doctor before embarking on a program. And anyone with impaired circulation to the legs and feet should find out what precautions to take. Dr. Peter Lodewick, chief diabetologist specialist at the Diabetes Department of the Eye Foundation Hospital in Birmingham, Alabama, says that such people should be particularly wary of getting blisters.

On a more encouraging note, we'd like to add that diabetes is no detriment to becoming an outstanding athlete. Some good examples are the tennis star Bill Talbert, the hockey player Bobby Clarke, and, in baseball, Jackie Robinson, Ron Santo, Bill Gullickson, and Catfish Hunter.

What kind of exercise should I do?

What kind of exercise do you like? Exercise should be fun. That's the only way to be sure you'll keep doing it. As a diabetic you have enough chores in your life without turning exercise into another one.

If you want to rate exercises, though, the ones that are best for you are the aerobic or endurance kind: brisk walking, jogging, running, swimming, cross-country skiing, biking (either on the real thing or, in bad weather, on an exercycle), rowing, jumping rope. Dancing is also a wonderful endurance exercise. There are now lots of aerobics classes designed especially to build up your cardiovascular system and endurance. Several television shows can lead you through a regular aerobic session, and you can buy videotapes to do the same.

But really, as we said, exercise is play and should be fun. Try to acquire a skill you enjoy, like tennis or bowling or golf, even if it isn't an endurance sport. We find that if you get really involved in a nonendurance sport, you tend to do some endurance exercising in order to—what else?—increase your endurance for the sport you love.

Yoga is also a wonderful exercise to keep you supple, and it's something that can be done at any age.

Be sure also to add to your activities some form of strengthening exercises. These are advocated by most experts now, because 60 percent of the body's muscles are above the hips. You can go a couple of times a week to a gym or fitness center (these also have aerobic equipment) and use Nautilus or Cybex strengthening equipment. Or simply work out at home with some weights.

You should have a minimum of three aerobic sessions a week of twenty to thirty minutes. Don't let more than two days elapse between workouts. It's better to exercise five times a week, and to our minds, exercising every day is the best, unless your body tells you not to, because then it's easier to balance your diet and medication. Incidentally, your blood sugar should be at least 150 before you begin your routine or you should eat a snack.

Your intensity goal should be to get your heart rate to between 60 and 65 percent of its maximum capacity. To figure your training pulse range, subtract your age from 220, then multiply the result by 60 percent. The 60 percent level is sufficient to promote fitness.

Before you begin an exercise program—and this is critical if you're out of shape—you should consult your physician and possibly have an exercise stress test. Your doctor may want to prescribe your individual heart target zone. And there is one instance in which exercise is harmful. If your blood sugar is 250 or over, exercise will simply run it higher and you may produce ketones.

The best time to exercise is after meals. This way, if you take insulin or oral drugs, you're less likely to get hypoglycemic. In fact, testing before, during, and after exercise is not a bad idea until you learn your blood-sugar pattern. You may need to lower your insulin or oral drug dosage or eat extra carbohydrate. Exercise has an effect on blood sugar for twenty-four hours. So watch for hypoglycemia (low blood sugar) the day after the exercise if you've done something special like a long hike or a day of skiing.

Type 1's should not inject insulin into the parts of the body that will be most used during exercise. For instance, don't inject into your legs or the arm you'll use if you're going to play tennis. The insulin would be absorbed much faster than usual if you did.

Incidentally, don't let age stop you. Even if you have health problems in addition to diabetes, there is always some form of exercise you can practice. Almost everyone can at least start walking on a schedule and then increase distance and speed until it becomes an endurance exercise.

As well as getting into a regular exercise program and sports, it's important to bring more exercise into your daily life simply by becoming a more physically active person. Get up out of your chair and move whenever possible. Climb stairs rather than taking the elevator. Park your car in the farthest corner of the parking lot and walk to the store. (Since everybody else is always trying to get as close as possible, you'll get the dividend of not having your car dinged up by the other people opening their doors on it.)

Is joining a gym a good way to get exercise?

It can be if you really go and go regularly. If you are gregarious and like to work out in the company of others, a gym may be just the motivation you need. It's a good way to get acquainted with people who have the same interest in fitness that you do. You can inspire one another— and chide one another when you don't show up. Be sure to join a gym that's not too far from your home, though, or you'll wind up spending most of your exercise time on transportation or decide not to go at all.

Belonging to a gym also has the advantage of providing someone to watch over you when you exercise. It is important to tell people there that you're a diabetic and to explain what the symptoms of hypoglycemia are so they can spot them in the event that you develop low blood sugar from exercise.

We heard peripatetic radio guru Bruce Williams say on one of his shows that when he belonged to a gym and got home from a trip, it was often too late to go to the gym or he was too tired to drive there, so he got himself a Schwinn Airdyne—an exercycle that exercises your arms as well as your legs. He said that when he got home "that darn thing was always there waiting for me and I had no excuses not to exercise." Purchasing your own exercise equipment and having it right at home might be a viable alternative for you. You could buy a new piece of equipment every year at about the cost of joining a gym. If there are others in your household who could use the equipment, it makes it an even better deal. Don't worry if you don't have a place to put it. Exercise equipment is getting more compact and portable all the time. We have a friend who keeps her rowing machine behind the sofa in the living room. Barbara has a treadmill, a rebounder, and a rowing machine in her bedroom. This doesn't leave much space for anything else, and it doesn't enhance the decor, but health is more important than decor any day.

Walking is, of course, one of the best exercises of all, and it takes no equipment. It does have a few drawbacks, though: you can't do it in all weather, and in big cities the streets and parks are getting acutely hazardous, especially for women alone. For these reasons mall-walking is becoming a popular alternative.

So analyze yourself and choose whatever would be most likely to keep you exercising regularly. Then just do it. (P.S.: *Do it now.*)

What should I do if I'm always too tired to exercise?

To some extent, that depends on what you did to get tired. If you're weary from your job as steeplejack or longshoreman, or if you're a housewife who's cleaned the whole house or galloped after a four-year-old all day, you've already had a great deal of exercise. Getting more is not that critical for you.

On the other hand, if you're tired from a long day of sedentary office tensions or sitting in the car, you need exercise for more reasons than diabetic ones, and you should clamp your jaw and force yourself, at least initially. Just as the appetite comes with the eating, the energy and enthusiasm for exercise come with the exercising. Often the fatigue you feel at the end of the day comes from a *lack* of physical activity rather than from too much of it.

If you find yourself too tired to exercise and it's not a true physical tiredness, you may go to bed and find yourself too keyed up and tense to sleep. The next day you've got a lack-of-sleep tiredness going. Vicious cycle. But if you get out there and move those bones around, blessed sleep will descend upon you as soon as you hit the pillow. You'll sleep the sleep of the physically tired and virtuous. And you can hardly sleep a better sleep than that.

Will vitamins and minerals help my diabetes?

For many years now we have always worn kid gloves and hip boots when exploring the vitamin/mineral jungle. If anything, the subject has gotten more controversial over the years, with Americans now being accused of having "vitamania." One hundred million of us are now spending $6.5 billion a year on vitamin and mineral pills. Of course, people with diabetes have more reason than most to be taking dietary supplements, as the FDA calls them, because their diets are often limited; and, as Dr. Richard Bernstein points out, high blood sugar causes excessive urination, and that results in the loss of water-soluble vitamins and minerals. But many R.D.'s and M.D.'s who specialize in diabetes tend to downplay the value of vitamins and minerals and refer to them as "hype without scientific evidence" and "no more than a way to get expensive urine."

So what's a poor diabetic to do? The soundest advice we can give you is to take at least one multiple vitamin/mineral pill a day as a good safety net. Diavite Plus with Antioxidants, which was formulated especially for people with diabetes, is available from Jordan Medical Enterprises of Garden Grove, California (call 1-800-342-8483). If you are on a high-fiber and/or high-protein diet, a calcium supplement is especially important because both fiber and protein bind calcium and cause a reduction in absorption. In his book Dr. Bernstein says, "I recommend calcium citrate (Citracal from Mission Pharmacal) because it is well absorbed in the gut and unlike other calcium formulations does not predispose to formation of kidney stones. Each tablet contains 315 mg. of elemental calcium. Appropriate daily doses are 2–6 tablets for men and 4–8 tablets for women. Calcium supplements should be taken with meals."

Two minerals often mentioned as having a positive effect on diabetes are zinc and chromium. Zinc plays a role in carbohydrate metabolism. Chromium deficiency can raise blood glucose while chromium supplementation can improve glucose tolerance in older people. At present there is no definitive evidence on the true value of taking these minerals unless you have a known deficiency. On the negative side, the Federal Center for Disease Control and Prevention found in a large study that zinc can impair immune responses and decrease your "good cholesterol."

What do we personally do? We take the multiple vitamin pills and we follow the current orthodoxy of the antioxidants C and E and the amount of calcium supplement advised for women of our ages plus even more to cover our high-fiber and high-protein diet. We neither condemn nor hype vitamins and minerals, but we do believe in the strong possibility of their therapeutic and preventive value depending on each of you finding the kind and dosage appropriate for your own health. It's another of those myriad personal-choice-with-the-guidance-of-your-health-care-team that people with diabetes are subject to.

And finally, we're glad you asked "Will vitamins and minerals *help* my diabetes?" and not "Will vitamins and minerals *cure* my diabetes?" We, too, have read, in books of vitamin lore, fables of how diabetics

were able to give up insulin injections entirely after loading up on vitamin supplements and health foods. Don't give yourself false hope. If
you have surplus money, it's better to give it to research for a real cure
for diabetes than to the vitamin industry for a false one.

What kind of eye problems can diabetes cause?

Blurred vision is one of the symptoms of long-term, out-of-control diabetes. After the diabetes is diagnosed and brought under control, vision usually returns to normal.

Because of the visual changes that can take place with changes in
blood sugar, June's ophthalmologist always insists that she have normal
blood sugar when she comes in to have her eyes checked to see if she
needs new glasses.

When a diabetic suddenly has blurred vision or other strange visual happenings (June sometimes reports seeing a large spot of light in
her field of vision), this can indicate low blood sugar. These changes in
vision can be disturbing, but they don't mean you're going blind. Blindness is always a worry for diabetics because you hear so many horren-
dous statistics about it. Diabetes used to be the cause of blindness in 11
percent of the legally blind people in this country, making it the third
leading cause of blindness. It is still the number-one cause of new cases
of blindness in people under sixty-five.

The culprit in diabetic blindness is retinopathy. This is a damaging of the blood vessels in the retina, the light-sensitive area in the back
of the eye. In its later stages the delicate blood vessels of the retina may
develop tiny sacs that can burst and leak blood, causing a loss of vision.

This is one of the reasons your doctor always examines your eyes
so carefully: to look for changes in your blood vessels. The retina is the
one place in the human body where doctors can actually see and inspect
the condition of the blood vessels. Not only is weakness in the walls of
the retinal blood vessels bad news in itself, but the condition of these
blood vessels reflects the condition of the vessels throughout the body.

You see, eyes are not just the mirrors of the soul, as the poets say, but the mirrors of the body as well.

Retinopathy is one of the diabetic horribles that doesn't have to happen. The study published in February 1989 in *JAMA* showed that no diabetic who had good control (less than 1.1 times normal blood sugar) had *any* eye damage, whereas of those who had blood sugar consistently above 1.5 times normal, 37 percent had retinopathy. The DCCT confirmed this.

Even when retinopathy does develop, all is not lost. There has been a great deal of success in treating it with laser beams. As always, however, the best treatment is to keep your blood sugar normal and not develop the problem in the first place.

Why do they talk so much about diabetic foot care?

It's that same old vascular story. Diabetes can cause hardening and narrowing of the blood vessels. This, in turn, causes poor circulation of the blood. Since the feet are farthest away from the great blood pump, the heart, they get the worst deal. Poor blood circulation is also part of the aging process. So if you're older *and* diabetic, you've really got to watch those feet.

And we do mean *watch,* because if you also have a touch of neuropathy, you may not feel a cut, sore, blister, or ingrown toenail and let it go until it becomes infected. Infections are particularly hazardous because, combined with diminished circulation, they provide a welcome mat for gangrene (tissue destruction), which can necessitate amputation.

Here are the foot-care dos:

1. Wash your feet every day and wear clean socks.
2. Always dry well between your toes.
3. Cut your toenails after bathing, following the shape of the ends of the toes. Do not cut too short.

4. Wear well-fitting shoes.
5. Examine your feet daily for signs of infection.
6. If you develop foot problems, go to a podiatrist and tell him or her you are diabetic. In fact, we favor regular visits to a podiatrist.

Here are the foot-care don'ts:

1. Avoid elastic garters or anything tight around the legs or ankles.
2. Do not use heating pads or hot-water bottles on your feet.
3. Avoid smoking; it reduces the blood supply to the feet.
4. Never walk around barefoot.
5. Do not use corn plasters or any over-the-counter foot medications.
6. Do not cut corns and calluses.
7. Do not put your feet in water warmer than 85 or 90 degrees Fahrenheit.

If you need convincing to make you behave yourself in the foot department, the Loma Linda Diabetes Education Program offers the story of a man who didn't take care of his diabetes *or* his feet. As he aged and deteriorated, he lost his sight and all feeling in his feet. Well, it came to pass that one night, without knowing it, he knocked his watch off his bedside table and into his shoe and broke the crystal. He walked around on said broken watch for two weeks. Needless to say, he wound up as a guest in the Loma Linda Hospital.

If you are a middle-aged or older diabetic, you should watch for symptoms of diminished circulation: weak pulses in the feet and legs; cold, dry, pale skin on the feet and legs; lack of hair growth on the toes; and toes that turn a dusky red color when they hang down, as when you're sitting on the edge of the bed. Be sure to mention it to your doctor if you notice any of these symptoms.

It is possible to improve or maintain the circulation in your feet with a simple exercise. Lie on a bed with your feet raised above your hips. Alternate pointing your toes and heels toward the ceiling. Do this several times. Make circles with your feet, first clockwise, then counterclockwise. Sit up with your feet hanging over the edge of the bed. Repeat the same maneuvers just described. Do this exercise a couple of times a day.

When you get your feet in good shape, walking a mile or more daily in comfortable shoes (runners' training shoes are good) can be of great benefit.

We don't want to give the impression that older diabetics are the only ones who have to be careful of their feet. Although younger people generally have better circulation, they still can get into trouble, especially if their diabetes is out of control.

Is there anything special I should do about my teeth?

If you're under good control, you'll treat your teeth as everyone is supposed to—daily flossing at night, brushing away the plaque at gum level after meals, regular visits to your dentist for removal of tartar (hardened plaque), and any other routines recommended for you personally. But if you have continual high blood sugars, your mouth, especially your gums, will be in jeopardy. The sad truth is that diabetes is sometimes diagnosed by a dentist because its damaging effects show up in your mouth.

What the dentist may see when inspecting the teeth of an individual who has undiagnosed or uncontrolled diabetes is periodontal (gum) disease. This is an inflammation of the gums and bone around the teeth caused by bacteria. Plaque is a soft accumulation of this bacteria. Plaque makes your gums bleed and eventually pull away from your teeth, forming open pockets that can deepen until you lose teeth.

Diabetes also lowers your mouth's ability to deter the bacterial infection. Bleeding gums are a sign of periodontal problems, as is bad breath. It pays, though it's expensive, to go to your dentist regularly, because periodontal disease and other oral infections can make blood-sugar control more difficult. It's the old vicious circle.

I have pain in my feet. My doctor says this is neuropathy. What is neuropathy?

Since the first edition of this book in 1981 we have received more letters about this complication of diabetes than any other. Simply put, neuropathy is nerve damage caused by high blood glucose. The most common type is "peripheral neuropathy," which means it affects the nerves in the feet, legs, and hands. Feet are the main source of complaint for most people.

The symptoms of neuropathy are described as pins and needles, tingling, numbness, or burning pain. You can even have complete loss of sensation. When this happens to your feet, it's very dangerous, because you won't be aware of blisters or injuries, or even of stepping on a tack.

Another form of neuropathy, "autonomic," affects the internal organs—stomach, urinary tract, small blood vessels, and even the genitals (this can cause impotence in men). Though generally not painful, this kind of nerve damage leads to serious disorders with the digestion (gastroparesis or slow emptying of the stomach), diarrhea or constipation, and unawareness of insulin reactions.

Treatments for all types of neuropathies start with bringing blood sugar under control. This alone can reverse the damage by as much as 50 percent in beginning cases. The strange phenomenon is that sometimes at first your discomfort becomes greater and lessens only after several months of normal blood sugars.

In cases of severe pain and gastrointestinal problems your doctor can prescribe various drugs. For peripheral neuropathy a cream called Zostrix or the three-times-stronger Axsain have proven effective for many people, but they often have to be used regularly for several weeks before you notice any improvement. Both these creams contain capsaicin, derived from chili peppers, so keep your fingers away from your eyes after applying it.

Researchers are now studying the use of a family of drugs called aldose-reductase inhibitors to treat mild cases of neuropathy. If the clinical trials are successful, these drugs may be of great benefit to sufferers.

Why do they say people with diabetes heal much more slowly than normal?

They say that because they don't differentiate between people in control (mostly normal blood sugars) and those out of control (mostly high blood sugars). If you are an in-control person, don't let health professionals prejudice you against yourself in this way. This is what Deepak Chopra, M.D., author of *Quantum Healing,* calls a *nocebo,* a term that denotes the opposite effect of a placebo. A nocebo is a negative effect caused by a doctor's opinion or prediction. If in a doctor's office you are told, "You won't heal very fast because of your diabetes," block out that thought, and if you have a good A_1C, tell yourself instead that your healing time will be normal or faster.

Testimonial: June once had a hand surgery (nothing to do with diabetes) and the orthopedic surgeon volunteered the statement, "You healed faster than most people."

Is it all right to use hot tubs?

According to the U.S. Consumer Product Safety Commission, all people who have diabetes, a history of heart disease, or blood-pressure problems should check with a doctor on the advisability of using a hot tub.

They also caution that nobody should bathe in a hot tub with water that is 104 degrees Fahrenheit or higher, since water of 106 degrees Fahrenheit can be fatal even to fully healthy adults. (Barbara, who considers herself a fully healthy adult, gets rather frightening nosebleeds after sitting in Japanese baths or hot springs.)

The preceding section on foot care explains that you shouldn't put your feet in water warmer than 85 or 90 degrees Fahrenheit. Since it's a little awkward to soak in a hot tub with your feet hanging out, it looks as if tepid tubs should be the order of the day for diabetics.

I have a bad case of acne. Could this be caused by my diabetes?

Possibly. Some diabetics report that they have acne when their diabetes is out of control and that it clears up when their blood sugar is stabilized.

Then again, it's possible that your acne has nothing to do with your diabetes. Many diabetics have a tendency to figure that every physical problem from acne to Zenker's diverticulum of the esophagus is related to their diabetes. When June had chronic headaches, she at first thought they were caused by low blood sugar. It turned out they had nothing to do with diabetes.

It is true that diabetes, especially out-of-control diabetes, can cause a variety of minor and not-so-minor health problems. Still, you should try to avoid laying the blame for everything on diabetes. Not only does this make you feel more depressed and put upon, but it may also cause you to delay seeking treatment for whatever your problem really is.

Are flu shots necessary?

They don't always work because there are often so many different strains of flu going around that you get zapped by one your shot doesn't cover. Still, we think they're a good idea. Flu can upset control of blood sugar for insulin takers, and flu shots are usually recommended for older people. Put those two groups together and you've just about covered the whole diabetic population.

Since flu shots themselves can cause rather heavy flu symptoms in susceptible beings, it's sometimes wise to take two half doses at different times. June always does this with flu shots and with shots she has to take for foreign travel as well.

Why do doctors always insist that you give up smoking?

Smoking is dangerous for everyone, but doubly dangerous for diabetics. Inhaling cigarette smoke affects the blood vessels. Diabetes can affect the blood vessels. Both diabetes and smoking tend to narrow them, and narrowed arteries can cause heart disease and gangrene.

An out-of-control diabetic has 2.5 times the normal chances of getting heart disease. A smoker has 1.7 times the normal chances of dying of heart disease. Put the two together and you have over 4 times the normal risk of heart disease.

An out-of-control diabetic has 60 times the normal chances of getting gangrene of the feet. Again, smoking increases that already dismal figure.

A study done at the University Hospital in Copenhagen, Denmark, found that diabetic patients who smoked required 15 to 20 percent more insulin than nonsmokers. Their level of blood fats was also higher.

You might call smoking a kind of Virginia roulette for diabetics. So why are there diabetic smokers? That's a question we have no answer for, except that their use of nicotine is an addiction harder to kick than an addiction to heroin. So people try and fail and try and fail ad infinitum.

The best suggestion we have is to seek help. Without help, your chance of quitting (and not relapsing) is slim indeed. A government survey found that only about 10 percent of the smokers who want to quit seek help. That is thought to be the reason why so few succeed.

Where can you get help? Many hospitals now have clinics or treatment centers specializing in smoking-cessation programs. There are independent programs too, like Smokenders and Schick. Ask your doctor for advice. Just be sure the system you try addresses all the dependency problems of smoking: the physical, the psychological, and the social. As Dr. Judith Ockene, director of preventive and behavioral medicine at the University of Massachusetts Medical Center, pointed out in a *New York Times* article, "the most effective methods deal with a smoker's three-pronged dependency and recognize that quitting is a process—not a one-time event—that occurs three or four times over five to ten years."

DIABETES AND YOUR DAILY LIFE

Should I tell people I have diabetes?

In general, definitely yes. You should tell everyone you have any kind of regular, everyday contact with—your hairdresser or barber, your colleagues at work, your teachers, your coaches, your friends (even rather casual ones), and especially those with whom you play sports.

You should make it a special point to tell anyone with whom you have any kind of medical and semimedical dealings, such as your dentist or podiatrist or oculist, because that may influence their treatment of you.

There are several good reasons for letting people know you have diabetes, especially if you are insulin-dependent. In the first place, should you have an insulin reaction, a person in the know can help you out or at least will realize that whatever is happening to you may be related to your diabetes and will get you to someone who can help.

You are also much less likely to inadvertently offend people if they know you have diabetes. For example, if you get low blood sugar and suddenly turn into a grouch or hellion, they may realize it's because of your diabetes, not because of a mean streak that's part of your nature. Then, too, if you're eating at a friend's house and turn down a sugar-shot confection, the cook will know that you're not insulting his or her culinary talents but just behaving yourself and dutifully following your own diabetic diet.

Another reason for informing people about your diabetes is that you can help out others by educating nondiabetics as to what diabetes is. What those with diabetes need is an each-one-teach-one program in order to spread diabetes facts and wipe out some of those weird fictions that are floating around in the public mind, such as, "People with diabetes can't eat sugar, but they can eat all the honey they want because honey is natural."

If you do tell others about your diabetes, you're also likely to find that you are not as alone in your condition as you thought. Almost everyone you mention your diabetes to will start telling you about a diabetic cousin or grandmother—or even about their diabetic selves!

As part of your diabetes announcement program, you should certainly wear some sort of identification bracelet or medallion. This is a safeguard in case you are ever in an accident or have some kind of diabetic problem when you're away from those who know you. A particularly good identification is a Medic Alert bracelet (available from Medic Alert Foundation, Turlock, California, 95381-1009, 1-800-ID ALERT). Medic Alert is well known now, and ambulance attendants, members of the ski patrol, and nurses in emergency hospitals are on the lookout for its insignia.

Now, after advocating this policy of extreme honesty, we'll hedge a bit. You don't have to be obsessed with your diabetes and immediately tell everyone you meet, "Hello-there-I'm-John-Smith-and-I'm-diabetic-pleased-to-meet-you," any more than you'd announce to a new acquaintance that you have gallstones or are colorblind or wear a pacemaker. As you get to know people better, your diabetes will emerge appropriately and naturally as a subject for conversation.

As for telling prospective employers and insurance agents, it's a yes-and-no situation that we'll discuss shortly.

Which is the correct thing to say: "I am a diabetic" or "I have diabetes"?

Do you mean correct or *politically* correct? Actually either is correct. As Lois Jovanovic-Peterson, M.D., wrote in *The Diabetic Woman,* "I always say that it doesn't matter if I am a person with syphilis or a syphilitic—I still have the same disease." The same holds true with diabetes. Several years ago *Diabetes in the News* ran a reader survey to see which was the preferred way. "I am a diabetic" won a clear victory. Most people thought it was more straightforward and more accepting of your condition.

But then was then and times have changed. If you want to be politically correct now, that's a different matter. There's a growing movement to never use "diabetic" as a noun. The ADA forbids its use in any of its publications. (On the other hand, we heard a radio ad for the Juvenile Diabetes Foundation in which they referred to "diabetics.")

We frequently get letters from people who range from wounded to furious when they're called "a diabetic." They feel that saying "I am a diabetic" gives the disease primary importance in your life, whereas saying "I have diabetes" or referring to "a person with diabetes" shows the disease to be of only secondary importance. Your individual personhood is what counts. And they certainly have a point.

June, call-a-spade-a-spade person that she is, has always referred to herself as "a diabetic," and you can see from the title of this book and the frequent reference to "diabetics" that we use the term interchangeably with the other more acceptable forms. But we don't like to gratuitously offend or hurt people to whom what they're called and call themselves makes a big difference. We tried to get the publisher to change the title of this book to *The Diabetes Book: All Your Questions Answered,* but that didn't fly because this is a new edition of a previously published book and you can't change the title in midstream.

And, although you may not believe it when you see the number of times we still use "diabetic and diabetics" as nouns in this new edition, we *have* made a concerted effort to be more sensitive to those who are offended by that usage. It's just that in order to keep the cost of production of the book (and, therefore, the price to the consumer) down, we weren't always able to change "diabetic" into "person with diabetes" when there were no other substantive changes to be made on that page or where there just wasn't space for the extra two words.

The pendulum, however, may be swinging back. In July 1993 the National Federation of the Blind adopted a resolution (#93-01) condemning all euphemisms for "blind" ("people with blindness," "visually impaired") and declaring that it is respectable to be blind and there is no shame in it.

But whether you use the approved or unapproved diabetes term, either will make you easily understood. Just don't shy away from both terms and use something cryptic the way June did once on a flight to Hawaii, when she was trying to get her meal from the flight attendant. "I'm on insulin," she said. "Could you serve me first?" The answer was negative. The problem, we figured out later, was that the flight attendant, who was Danish, didn't have any idea what June was talking about. In fact, she probably thought that insulin was the name of some kind of group tour of the islands and that June was just trying to get a special privilege for no good reason.

When Barbara trotted back a few minutes later and made eyeball-to-eyeball contact with the flight attendant and announced, "My friend is a di-a-bet-ic" (that's the way she said it back in those days!) "and she needs to eat. Could you serve her now?" the meal appeared a few seconds faster than immediately.

Now on to the question of the grammar of the words *diabetic* and *diabetes*. Experts have very definite ideas about correctness in the use of the words *diabetes* and *diabetic*. They don't like you to use *diabetic* as an adjective, unless what you're talking about actually has diabetes. For example, "The diabetic man had a diabetic dog" is all right, because both the man and the dog are diabetics. "The diabetic education lecture was held at the diabetic study center" is all wrong, because neither the education lecture nor the study center has diabetes. It should be "The diabetes education lecture was held at the diabetes study center."

You wouldn't say "a diabetic specialist" unless the specialist you're talking about has diabetes. If he's a specialist in diabetes, he should be called a diabetes specialist. If he's a specialist in diabetes who has diabetes, then presumably he'd be referred to as a "diabetic diabetes specialist." But maybe you think this is being linguistically nitpicky. Maybe we think so, too.

Just to put the capper on the whole nomenclatural confusion, the British call their organization the British Diabetic Association. But they always did have trouble with the language.

Will I be able to get insurance?

That depends on the kind of insurance you're interested in getting.

Automobile insurance. There should be no trouble if you're in good control. (Here's yet another reason to take good care of yourself.) If they ask on the form if you're a diabetic, naturally you have to tell them. In that case, they'll probably ask you to produce a letter from your doctor saying that your diabetes is under control.

If they don't ask, we don't see any point in saying, "Hey there, insurance company, I have diabetes. Don't you want to hassle me?" Personal experience: June's automobile insurance company has never asked; she has never told.

Life insurance. If you're in control (again, with evidence required) and you take less than forty units of insulin—or don't take insulin at all—you should have no more difficulty getting life insurance than a nondiabetic. We have, however, heard of cases in which people working for very small companies were denied both life insurance and disability insurance coverage on company policies.

Health insurance. We don't need to tell you that this a major problem fraught with confusion as far as people with diabetes are concerned. Without good health insurance or a government entitlement, it's almost impossible to take the best care of yourself, unless your name is Donald Trump, Bill Gates, or Oprah Winfrey (none of whom has diabetes). Choosing the best possible plan available to you is of crucial importance, and the health care insurance industry has become a confusing maze with Gorgons waiting for you at every turn. It's a consumer-beware world out there, but there is some good news, especially for those on Medicare.

Although there are more unknowns than knowns in what the future holds for health insurance in America, one thing is pretty certain. More and more people will be with health maintenance organizations (HMOs) than ever before. These are the least expensive choice in health insurance. In California more than 90 percent of those with insurance are enrolled in some form of managed care (another name for HMOs and the like), and this reflects the national trend. The problem with HMOs for diabetics is that they are the most restrictive plans, in that they limit your choice of doctors and generally require that you get approval from a "gatekeeper" (some say they act more like hockey goalies!) or your primary care doctor for approval to receive certain services or be referred to a specialist. In fact, here's a little joke that appeared in the *Los Angeles Times* "Laugh Lines" column: "An Apparition a Day Keeps the Doctor Away: A poll says 94 percent of HMO executives believe spirituality can help cure illness. They'll try anything that doesn't involve a referral to a specialist."

Health maintenance organizations claim that they pay more for preventive health services than other types of health plans, and many of them do have educational services such as weight management and, in some plans, diabetes education. Before signing up for an HMO plan it's most important for you to find out if it will pay for your diabetes supplies and what the limitations are. As you can see from the following table, which appeared in *Diabetes Interview,* the kind of intensive diabetes therapy recommended by the DCCT to prevent complications is expensive. The next least expensive option is a preferred-provider organization (PPO). With these you must go to a doctor in the approved network, and even then you pay a small amount for your office visit. You can see a doctor who does not belong to the PPO, but you'll pay more in out-of-pocket costs.

DIABETES INTERVIEW ESTIMATE

TREATMENT METHOD	CONVENTIONAL THERAPY (using injections)	INTENSIVE THERAPY (using multiple injections)	INTENSIVE THERAPY (using an insulin pump)
Shots/Day	2	4	Continuous
Insulin & syringe or infusion set	44¢	88¢	$3.66
pump cost/day	—	—	$2.67
Blood Tests/Day	2	8	8
Strip Cost (72¢ ea.)	$1.44	$5.80	$5.80
Supply Cost/Month	$101	$247	$368.96
Supply Cost/Year	$1,208*	$2,960*	$4,427.45*

*Includes $125 meter, cost spread over two years. Pump therapy includes $3,900 pump, cost spread over four years.
(Reprinted from *Diabetes Interview*. For more information call 1-800-473-4636.)

The most expensive form of health insurance is the traditional plan, which gives you total freedom, but the cost of joining can be very high (say $5,000 a year) unless you can participate as part of a large group (a company or professional organization, for instance).

Medicare. The bright note on the diabetes health insurance scene is that beginning July 1, 1998, Medicare will reimburse for blood-glucose meters and test strips for all patients with diabetes, not just for those who take insulin as it was before. Medicare will also cover self-management education programs that have achieved ADA Recognition status. Another breakthrough has been that fourteen more states have enacted laws that require reimbursement for diabetes education and supplies by state-regulated health insurance companies, bringing the total to twenty-three states. The states that have passed diabetes health insurance reforms as of 1998 are: Arkansas, Connecticut, Florida, Indiana, Louisiana, Maine, Maryland, Minnesota, Missouri, New Hampshire, New Jersey, New Mexico, New York, Nevada, North Carolina, Oklahoma, Rhode Island, Tennessee, Texas, Vermont, Washington, West Virginia, and Wisconsin.

Both state governments and the federal government are finally stepping in to restrict the way HMOs operate and to prevent them from putting restraints on good care. There is a movement to establish a patient "bill of rights" for consumer protection. There are proposals to allow patients to appeal denials of treatment, to have appropriate access to emergency services, and to allow participation in treatment decisions and a broad-enough choice of doctors and providers to ensure quality care. Watch newspapers and magazines for the latest developments so that you can take advantage of them.

A very good book to consult is *Managing Diabetes on a Budget* by Leslie Y. Dawson. Published in 1995 by the ADA, it explains how to get the most out of your insurance coverage and offers other tips on cost-saving ways to manage diabetes. (See the reference section.)

Will diabetes keep me from getting a job?

It didn't keep actress Mary Tyler Moore, radio and TV personality Gary Owens, hockey star Bobby Clarke, prominent physician Peter Forsham, or McDonald's restaurant tycoon Ray Kroc from getting the jobs they wanted. Why would it keep you from any career you choose? The truth is that the great majority of people with diabetes have the same employment opportunities and limitations as nondiabetics. So if you're qualified for a particular position, go after it positively and aggressively, and with confidence. Studies have shown that having diabetes promotes not only a healthy life-style but also great self-discipline. These in turn lead to superior performance on the job.

We have two examples of young men seeking their heart's choice of career—to be a doctor—in spite of being type 1 diabetics. Their experiences also demonstrate the difference between then and now, between the old days of prejudice and discrimination against diabetics and the new ones of open opportunity.

Then

George L. Chappell, M.D., a psychiatrist practicing in Ventura, California, has been a diabetic for over thirty-seven years now. He knew from the age of four that he wanted to be a physician, so he actually overqualified himself during high school and college: high grades, a job, community volunteer service, everything to show he could succeed and carry a heavy workload. He applied to twenty medical schools and was rejected by all of them. One admissions officer told him: "Well, George, your qualifications are certainly way above average, but you're not going to live long enough for society to regain the investment that it makes in your education, so we won't be able to accept you." But Dr. Chappell persisted, pulling every string he could until finally the admissions officer at the University of California at Los Angeles caved in. He is still very much alive and has found the struggle well worth it, as "the emotional and professional rewards are great." He says that because of diabetes, he has a degree of empathy and personal experience that physically healthy physicians lack. Many of his patients notice his special concern and are grateful to have found such an out-of-the-ordinary therapist.

Now

Our first employee at the original SugarFree Center in Van Nuys, California, Ron Brown, joined us the summer before he planned to enter a Ph.D. program in psychology. As a diabetic himself, he had an instant rapport with all of our clients and, because of his deep reading in the field of diabetes, was invaluable in providing support and counseling.

The warm feelings that our clients felt toward Ron were obviously reciprocated. He soon knew that he wanted to devote his life to working with diabetics. Because of his talent for gourmet cooking and because he saw the difficulty most diabetics have in understanding and adjusting to the dietary changes their disease requires, he decided to work toward his R.D. degree.

After his swift and successful completion of the R.D. program at the University of California at Berkeley, he came back to work with us at the Del Mar, California, SugarFree Center and served as a dietitian at the nearby Scripps Clinic. His increased experience in diabetes at Scripps and with us heightened his interest in the field and made him realize that to do as much as he wanted to do to help others with diabetes, he would have to become a physician. Therefore, on top of working both at Scripps and at the SugarFree Center, he took the additional premed courses he lacked.

Ron applied for entrance to medical school in 1986 at the age of thirty. Both his age and his diabetes could have worked against him. Neither did. He was accepted by three medical schools without a quibble and probably would have been accepted by more except that he withdrew his other applications when he was accepted at the one he really wanted, the University of California at Davis. He now has his M.D.

Not only does Ron's story show that prejudices against diabetes in the work world are crumbling, but it poses an interesting question. Would he be where he is today—getting ready to embark on a medical career—if he had not developed diabetes? As our former nurse-educator, Elsie Smallback, always said, "Out of something bad comes something good."

Ron's story reminds us of what we read about prize-winning novelist Walker Percy. He had gone to medical school because it was the thing to do in his family. After graduation he decided to go into psychiatry and interned at Bellevue Hospital in New York. He never practiced, though, because he contracted pulmonary tuberculosis and spent three years recuperating. For much of that time he was flat on his back, reading voraciously, mostly fiction and philosophy, which ultimately led to his literary career. He calls tuberculosis "the best disease I ever had. If I hadn't had it, I might be a second-rate shrink practicing in Birmingham at best."

Some years from now, it will be interesting for you to muse awhile on how your life has changed *for the better* because of your diabetes. You may well be surprised at what you come up with.

Realistic optimists that we are, however, we do have to report a few—very few—negatives in career selection for diabetics who take insulin. You should avoid jobs where you could endanger yourself or others during insulin reactions. It wouldn't be wise for you to seek jobs that involved high-speed machinery or climbing around on skyscraper construction girders, for example. Legally, there are certain restrictions, too. The federal government does not allow diabetics on insulin to enter the armed forces or to pilot airplanes. The Federal Highway Administration now allows type 1's and 2's on insulin to have commercial licenses to drive trucks and buses in interstate commerce. This is only if they are under a doctor's care and are not prone to seizures. However, a woman who had moved from New York to Florida and whose husband was insulin-dependent but had no episodes of hypoglycemia on his record reported to us that a clever lawyer representing a powerful company managed to get around this ruling, and her husband lost his job when they moved to Florida.

If you should run into job discrimination because of diabetes, don't hesitate to fight it. Federal regulations have made it illegal for most major employers to reject you solely because you have diabetes. The Americans with Disabilities Act, which considers diabetes legally a disability, gives you the option of filing a complaint if you experience discrimination in the workplace. Employers cannot even ask you if you have diabetes during a job interview and must make reasonable accommodation for your diabetes needs.

FOR MEN:
Will my diabetes cause sexual problems?

According to early statistics, between 40 and 60 percent of diabetic men are ultimately affected by impotence. (A variation on this statistical theme is that the incidence of impotence is 15 percent in diabetic men between the ages of thirty and forty and 55 percent by age fifty.) As Mark Twain said, "There are lies, damned lies, and statistics." These statistics are probably akin to the now false figures about how many diabetics go blind or have amputations and kidney failure—all computed from the period when we didn't have the therapies we now have to keep blood sugar normal.

We actually hate to even quote these impotence statistics since reading them is just the sort of thing that could cause it. One psychologist we heard at a conference recounted the story of one of his patients who wasn't aware of the existence of diabetic impotence and was getting along just fine. When he heard the discouraging word, it was instant impotence for him. So if you're not having any problems in that line and if you're keeping your blood sugar normal, forget the statistics and go on with your life—and your sex life. If you've had or are having some problems or harbingers thereof, read on.

First of all, the impotence legends reflect several factors. Sometimes when a man is an undiagnosed, out-of-control diabetic, he can develop a *temporary* impotence, which goes away when his diabetes is diagnosed and he gets his blood sugar back in the normal range. This has inflated the statistics just cited.

Second, when diabetes is first diagnosed, a man is shot with so many negative emotions—such as anxiety, depression, anger, guilt, fear of rejection, and worry over his future—that he becomes impotent for psychological reasons, not because of his diabetes.

Sometimes the problem is caused by what sex therapists William H. Masters and Virginia E. Johnson call "spectatoring." Raul C. Schiavi and Barbara Hogan, writing in *Diabetes Care,* vividly describe the situation in which a diabetic man has heard the statistics and wonders if he's going to be a victim of them: "The diabetic patient, rather than becoming involved in the sexual experience and abandoning himself into erotic sensations and feelings, may find himself constantly monitoring the state of his penis. He becomes a witness rather than a participant in the sexual experience." Not surprisingly, this "performance anxiety" often results in impotence.

Indeed, the *British Medical Journal* reported that diabetic impotence was most likely caused by psychological factors in two-thirds of the men studied and by physical factors in only one-third. On the other hand, the brochure of the Recovery of Male Potency Program at Grace Hospital in Detroit says, "Twenty years ago, most doctors thought that impotence was primarily a psychological problem. We now realize that 80 percent of impotence has a physical rather than a psychological cause." And Ginger Manley, R.N., M.S.N., writing in the *Diabetes Educator,* states, "While in the general population only about 50 percent of impotence is physical in origin, in the diabetic population physically mediated impotence approaches 90 percent." (You read your statistics and you take your choice.) In short, impotence can be a combination of physical and psychological factors.

An easy and inexpensive way for you to determine if impotence is psychological or physical has been suggested by the broadcaster-columnist Dr. Gabe Mirkin. He explains that there are two stages of sleep: rapid-eye-movement (REM) and non-rapid-eye-movement sleep. In non-rapid-eye-movement sleep, males achieve an erection. This can occur several times throughout the night, and the male wakes up the next morning without even knowing it happened.

If you are achieving erections in the night, your impotence is psychological. To check this out, Dr. Mirkin recommends taking a roll of postage stamps (the one-cent kind, for thrift's sake), tearing off the appropriate number of stamps (he suggests four), and securing them tightly to the penis before going to bed. If the stamps are torn apart in the morning, you know you're having erections.

To make sure that anxiety resulting in fitful sleep doesn't confuse the issue, it might be a good idea to try this test more than once before deciding that your impotence is physical rather than psychological.

What can I do about impotence that is mainly psychological?

We hope it will help some just to have the reassurance that it *is* mainly psychological and that when you start handling the negative emotions that engulfed you with your diagnosis of diabetes, the sex problem will gradually disappear.

We know, however, that such emotions and their effects can't always be swept away with logic and Dutch-uncle conversations with yourself. You can't immediately eliminate your problem just because you've been told what's causing it. It takes time and consideration (consideration of yourself by yourself as well as consideration from your partner). If it takes too much time—and only you can decide how much is too much—you shouldn't hesitate to get some psychological help.

If your doctor isn't able to recommend a psychological counselor or sex therapist, you can contact any large university in your area. Most of these have human-sexuality programs and can give you the names of qualified sex therapists who are available for private consultation. And it is imperative that both you and your partner go to the therapist.

What can I do about impotence that is caused by physical factors?

Richard K. Bernstein, M.D., in his book *Diabetes: The GlucograF™ Method for Normalizing Blood Sugar,* suggests that if impotence in type 1 diabetics is occasional and if it occurs during the first five to ten years of the disease, the "inability to become aroused or, if aroused, inability to achieve orgasm can be an early warning of hypoglycemia [low blood sugar]. . . . This early warning sign has been detected by both males and females. In fact, patients have located the blood-sugar levels at which they 'turn off.' " He continues, "It appears that both men and women tend to have two turnoff points: at one blood-sugar level they can be aroused but cannot achieve orgasm; at a lower blood-sugar level they cannot even be aroused. . . . Some patients try to prevent an unpleasant situation by measuring blood sugar when feasible prior to anticipated intercourse and promptly take fast-acting sweets if blood sugar is low."

You can also become impotent while under the influence of certain drugs. Among these are alcohol, tranquilizers, and marijuana. In many older men, impotence may be caused by hypertension drugs, with diabetes getting the blame. When possible, these suspect drugs should be avoided or their use discontinued. Your physician may be able to suggest an alternative medication.

Most long-range, gradually occurring impotence in diabetics is due to one or a combination of three factors:

1. a decrease in the male hormone, testosterone. This is the least likely of the three. It can be treated with hormone injections.
2. an interruption of the blood flow to the penis, usually as a result of atherosclerosis (hardening of the arteries).
3. neuropathy—damage to the nerves that carry the sexual message from the brain and dilate the blood vessels. This neuropathy is usually caused by long-term poor control of blood sugar and is sometimes reversible with improved control.

As for treatments, the simple-to-use breakthrough pill Viagra was approved by the FDA in March 1998. It is expected to work 70 percent of the time for erectile dysfunction.

Some other treatments that have proved successful include injections of drugs that improve the supply of blood to the penis, the use of vacuum-constriction devices, and penile implants. The implants can be rigid, semirigid, or inflatable. Anyone seeking help with physiological impotence should consult with a urologist. There are also many hospitals now setting up impotency programs where the problem of impotence can be evaluated, the options explained, and corrective procedures instituted. These programs often include invaluable support groups.

For background reading on diabetic impotence and its treatment, there is the "Sexual Man" chapter in the book *The Diabetic Man* by Peter Lodewick, M.D. There is also an excellent article, "Diabetes and Sexual Health," by Ginger Manley, R.N., M.S.N., in vol. 12, no. 4, of *The Diabetes Educator.* If you can't find it in a local library, write to the AADE (see the reference section).

It's important to remember that with impotence, as with all problems associated with diabetes, the best treatment is no treatment—that is to say, preventive maintenance that keeps the problem from developing in the first place. As Dr. Neil Baum, director of the New Orleans Impotence Foundation, says, "Men with poorly controlled diabetes have decreased sex drive as well as problems with impotence. Good control is associated with improvement in potency, libido, and sense of well-being."

FOR WOMEN:
Will my diabetes cause sexual problems?

Previously it had been thought that diabetes had little or no effect on either a woman's sexual performance or satisfaction. Even now, based on what diabetic women report to their doctors, it would seem that they reach a sexual climax just as often as nondiabetic women.

Still there are rumblings from some diabetes therapists—especially female diabetes therapists—that sex problems associated with diabetes are as common among women as among men. It's just that the male sex problems have been given more attention. This is not necessarily due to sexism. It may be due to the fact that sexual response is easier to measure with men than with women. (And easier for women to fake than men.)

The majority of women's sexual problems appear to be related to poor diabetes control. A woman understandably loses interest in sex when she is excessively tired and run down from being out of control. High blood sugar and the resulting sugar in the urine increase susceptibility to vaginal infections that cause swelling, itching, burning, and pain, which are hardly conducive to enthusiasm for sexual intercourse. These infections can be treated with salves (Monistat or Gyne-Lotrimin), but the only real cure is keeping your diabetes under control.

If a long-term diabetic woman develops neuropathy (damaged nerve cells)—again often as a result of poor control—it may involve the nerve fibers that stimulate the genitalia so that arousal may not occur, making intercourse painful because lubricating fluids are not released. Arthur Krosnick, M.D., writing in *Diabetes Forecast,* recommends the use of water-soluble lubricants, such as K-Y Lubricating Jelly, for this condition. He also states that "estrogen deficiency responds to vaginal creams. These creams are available by prescription and do not affect diabetes control."

Emotional factors associated with diabetes—anxiety, fear, anger, and, especially, depression—can significantly decrease a woman's desire for sex, especially since these negative emotions often result in (or are a result of) poor diabetes control.

Dr. Lois Jovanovic-Peterson, writing in *The Diabetic Woman,* neatly sums up the situation: "The best way to be sexy and enjoy sex, therefore, is to be happy, healthy, fit, and in good control of your blood-glucose levels."

She also offers this handy hint for insulin-taking diabetic women when things are going well in the sex department: "If a woman thoroughly enjoys the sexual encounter, the sheer exercise of the experience may result in a severe hypoglycemic episode. Thus, a woman needs to be prepared. She should adjust her insulin downward in anticipation of the evening, or if the evening happens to be on the spur of the moment, she should compensate by eating something afterward."
Bon appétit!

Should I become pregnant?

We assume from this question that you have already wrestled through the basic Everywoman life decision of whether to have children and have concluded that you want to, but you worry about the effect your diabetes will have on your baby and vice versa.

The first consideration is: Do you have any diabetes complications such as retinopathy (diabetic eye damage), neuropathy (nerve damage), or poor kidney function? If so, you may have to postpone the idea of becoming pregnant, because pregnancy could worsen the condition. Oddly enough, it can go both ways. In the case of retinopathy, Dr. Jovanovic-Peterson told us that "of one hundred women with retinopathy, 50 percent have no change, 25 percent get better, and 25 percent get worse with pregnancy." It is for this reason that before entering into a pregnancy you need to consult with your diabetes specialist to make sure you have a normal hemoglobin A_1C; with your gynecologist; with an ophthalmologist; and with a urologist.

If all systems are go, you can be cheered by the news that your chances of having a healthy baby are exactly the same as a nondiabetic woman's. The one great warning is to establish normal blood sugar (a normal A_1C) *before* becoming pregnant. Otherwise, you're in trouble from the start.

We must also forewarn you that a diabetic woman's pregnancy means a great intensification of self-care. Blood sugar must be monitored on a meter between five and ten times a day. Blood-sugar level must be kept between 60 and 90 before meals and less than 140 after meals during the entire term of the pregnancy. This means excessive risk of hypoglycemia for type 1's. That's why the pregnancy is sometimes harder on the husband than the wife. For a preview of your pregnancy and a view of what the regime is like, read "Happy, Healthy Babies: Type I Women" in *The Diabetic Woman,* 1996 edition (see the reference section).

Cost is also an important factor. The major expenses are blood-sugar-testing supplies and fetal monitoring (amniocenteses, ultra-sounds, fetal-echo checks, and fetal nonstress tests).

If your main concern involves the ethics of producing a child with the possibility of diabetic heredity, that's a decision only you can make. Fortunately, the pattern of inheritance of diabetes is now much clearer, and the picture looks brighter than it did just a few years ago. Children of type 1 diabetics have only a 2 to 6 percent chance of also becoming diabetic. Non-insulin-dependent diabetes is more inheritable. The children of type 2's have a 15 to 25 percent chance of becoming diabetic.

What is the best contraceptive for a woman to use?

Birth control for diabetic women is essentially the same as for nondiabetic women. The choice is up to the woman, her partner, and her gynecologist. The most commonly used method is the low-dose pill. A newer dosage form of "oral contraceptives" is Depo Provera, an injection. These pills are not considered dangerous unless you have high blood pressure or retinopathy. Ordinarily they do not have an impact on your insulin doses, but in higher dosages they can change insulin requirements, and thus it's best to keep in touch with your diabetes doctor and gynecologist about this.

The longstanding barrier methods are okay, also—diaphragms, condoms, and cervical sponges. For women who are certain they don't want to become pregnant in the future, sterilization (obviously) is the most reliable method.

One diabetic woman we talked to said she thinks the safest and most reliable method of contraception is a husband with a vasectomy.

And, finally, a previous editor, who felt we should present every possible option in this book, offered the reminder, "There's always celibacy."

Can people with diabetes travel?

Anyone who knows the two of us at all will realize that we would consider that question as ridiculous as asking "Can people with diabetes breathe?" Travel is that much a part of our lives—and we feel it should be that much a part of yours.

On this shrinking planet, your job may require you to travel all over the country or even all over dozens of other countries. Never let your diabetes stop you. If you keep yourself under good control and plan ahead, you'll make business trips with as much ease and success as the nondiabetic next person. As a matter of fact, because of your good health habits, you may well be brighter and more alert and ready for the work than nondiabetics, who may feel a little headachy from airline cocktails or drowsy from carousing.

Terrence Mason, a trainer for the Grantmanship Center in Los Angeles, spends an estimated 60 to 70 percent of his time traveling all over the world. In the Summer 1989 issue of *Living Well with Diabetes,* the quarterly journal published by the International Diabetes Center in Minneapolis, Minnesota, Mason says that because he is black he has to recognize that he may encounter prejudices and stereotyping in his travels and be prepared for them. Once when he needed to purchase syringes he found that because of his color he was automatically suspected of being a drug user. "I could go into places, as middle-class and as old as I am," he says, "and there'd be many places that just wouldn't sell me syringes." His doctor later explained that he could always go to a hospital emergency room and get syringes. But now he also carries his doctor's phone number so he can call to request that a prescription be prepared by another doctor in the city where he's traveling. That's a good idea for anyone of any color.

Carrying a letter from your doctor explaining that you have diabetes and outlining your treatment needs is also a good idea. This is not just to help you get syringes or insulin or whatever else you need in an emergency, but to identify you as a diabetic in case customs inspectors notice your syringes. This is especially true for young people; we know of one young woman on a school-sponsored educational tour who was interrogated by the authorities at one border because of her syringes. They wound up believing her, but it was a very disturbing experience for her because the whole tour group was held up while she was being worked over. It was an experience that could have been avoided with a doctor's letter and plenty of diabetes identification.

In the back of our now out-of-print book *The Peripatetic Diabetic,* we include identification information for insulin-taking diabetics in Danish, Dutch, Finnish, French, German, Greek, Italian, Japanese, Norwegian, Portuguese, Russian, Spanish, and Swedish. You can probably find a copy of this book in a library and copy whichever i.d.'s you need. If you can't locate a copy, call us at 1-800-735-7726 or e-mail prana 2@aol.com and we'll be happy to run off a copy of whatever you need and send it to you.

Even more important than business travel, though, is the travel you do for pleasure and mind expansion. To our way of thinking, the vacation spent puttering around the house is not a vacation at all. A true vacation gets you away from home and away from the routine demands on your time and the routine worries that constantly nibble on your subconscious.

The strange thing is that if you just get away for a short time— even a weekend—you feel so restored and unstressed that it's as if you'd had a month-long holiday.

If you're nervous about handling your diabetes away from home, you might try our "expanding circle" method of travel. Make your first trip a weekend jaunt to a very nearby town or, if you live in a large city, to another part of the same city. You can pretend you're on the opposite side of the earth, but you know you can get home fast or get in touch with your doctor if there's an emergency.

When you've proved to yourself that staying in a hotel and eating all your meals out poses no problems to you or your diabetes, expand the circle farther by going someplace about five hundred miles away.

Next travel all the way across the country to a place you've always wanted to visit. Then try Canada or Hawaii—both have a foreign feeling yet pose no language or food problems.

Finally, after you've had success in these areas, go to Europe or Asia or Australia or Africa or even Antarctica, if that's your pleasure. For the truth is that a diabetic can travel anywhere that diabetics live and, of course, that's every country on earth.

Now that you're all hyped up and ready to go, here are a few of our favorite travel tips and precautions.

- Take double quantities of all diabetes and other medical supplies that you use. It may not be easy to find them, especially overseas, and besides, who wants to spend vacation time shopping in pharmacies? If you're a belt-and-suspenders type, as June is, carry half your supplies in one place and half in another so that if you should lose a purse or piece of luggage, you'll still be covered. Then, just to be on the absolutely safe side, carry along a prescription for any medication you take. Have your doctor make this for the generic name of the drug, since the trade name may vary from country to country.

- Try to go to just one place. In the United States make it one city or national park or resort area; overseas, just one country. (A few years ago we actually went just to Rome for three weeks.) If you don't try to gulp down the whole world on a single vacation, you'll spend more time being there rather than going to a lot of different theres. You'll have more time on your feet exploring or playing than on your seat in a car or bus or train or plane. Your diabetes will show its appreciation. And if you go to only one country, you'll be able to do research ahead of time into the native cuisine to make your meals easier to figure, and more fun as well. You'll also be able to learn a few appropriate phrases in the language ("I am a diabetic." "Where is the restroom?" "Quick! Get me some sugar!").

- Sports vacations are wonderful. Not only do you get healthful and restoring exercise while you're there, but you can also take lessons to acquire (or hone) a skill like tennis or golf or skiing that will enrich you and make your whole life healthier.

- Two short vacations are better than one long one. You get the welcome release of a holiday at two different times of the year instead of just one. And it's true that it becomes wearisome to stay away from home for too long. June prefers vacations of one or two weeks, but if she's going overseas, she's willing to stretch it to three. Her basic rule: "I come home when all my clothes are dirty."

- Take along two pairs of broken-in (*not* broken-down) shoes. If possible, change your shoes in the middle of the day. This helps prevent blisters. Walk and walk and walk and walk. You'll see more and get to *eat* more that way.

- As you start your trip, make it a point to slip into what Olympic gold-medal marathon runner and attorney Frank Shorter calls his "travel mode." This means keeping relaxed and making a conscious effort not to let anything bother you. If there's a flight delay, no matter. If a crying baby is seated nearby, no matter. If someone whaps your ear with a flight bag when putting it in the overhead compartment, no matter. Remain in a semimeditative state, a kind of "serene mellowness," as Shorter puts it. Getting angry and upset over the inevitable annoyances associated with travel only hurts (and raises the blood sugar of) one person: you.

- Another Shorter travel tip is to be especially pleasant to any of the service people you deal with on a trip. He finds that courtesy is usually returned in kind and often serves to iron out potential wrinkles in your trip (and on your brow).

- Take all the normal precautions any prudent traveler—diabetic or not—would take. For example, be sure all your basic shots are up to date. Tetanus is a particularly important one because, in case of an accident, getting a tetanus shot on top of whatever other trauma you're experiencing just exacerbates the condition. If there's a flu going around, it usually goes around everywhere, so have a shot for that unless you've had one recently. You should check with your travel agent to see what extra shots are recommended for the places you're visiting and take those as well. Any shots you take should be taken well ahead of time. If you get a reaction to any of them, you don't want it to take place on the trip. Besides, it sometimes takes a while for the immunity to set in and keep you covered. Check to find out if your health insurance covers you in foreign countries; if it doesn't, talk to your travel or insurance agent about a special short-term policy to cover you while you're traveling.

- For foreign travel, write to the International Diabetes Federation, International Association Center, 40 Washington St., 1050 Brussels, Belgium; phone 32-2-647-41-14, for a list of diabetes specialists. You might also purchase membership in the International Association for Medical Assistance to Travelers (IAMAT) for a seventy-two-page directory of English-speaking doctors around the world. IAMAT's address: 417 Center St., Lewiston, NY 14092; phone 716-754-4883.
- Two other handy things to take with you on a trip: a small but bright-beamed flashlight so you won't stub your toe while stumbling around strange hotel rooms in the dark looking for the bathroom or your testing materials or snacks or whatever you might need during the night for your diabetes care (this will also come in handy for reading menus in dark restaurants); and a friend or relative who understands diabetes and can help you cope with the unexpected.
- Relax and have a good time.

Follow these rules and, indeed, the longest and most grueling of flights or bus, train, or car trips will seem shorter.

How can I get special diabetic meals on airplanes?

You can request them when you buy your tickets and the agent relays your order to the airline. If you later change your flight, you must inform the airline so that it can switch your meal order, too.

Virtually all airlines offer special diabetic trays. Once, however, when we flew United Airlines to Hawaii, the dietary-meal request slip was accidentally left on the tray. This showed that the same meal was being delivered to all those who had made these special requests for meals: diabetic, Hindu, Moslem, hypoglycemic, low calorie, low carbohydrate, low cholesterol, low fat, and low sodium. Clearly, a meal that tries to be appropriate for all of the above is not going to be totally right for any of them. And it wasn't. There was not a starch exchange to be found on the tray.

After years of trying on dozens of airlines, we've finally given up and now just take what comes. June can sort through it and pick out what she needs. After all, when immobilized on an airplane, a diabetic can eat very little anyway. It's better to concentrate not on food but rather on drinking lots of water (so you won't get dehydrated from the dry air in the cabin) and walking up and down the aisle as often as you can to keep your circulation chugging along. Drinking alcohol on a flight isn't too smart, either, since it, too, is dehydrating.

Naturally, you should bring along lots of snacks in case for some reason no food of any kind appears, or appears much later than you need it.

How can I avoid getting diarrhea when I travel in foreign countries?

Sometimes you can't. Each country has its own varieties of bacteria in the water and food. The very fact that these are different from the ones you're accustomed to causes the classic tourist problem.

Both type 1's and type 2's should, of course, do everything possible to protect themselves from diarrhea. In south-of-the-border countries where *turista* is a special threat, or overseas in less developed countries, drink only bottled water and avoid drinks containing ice. According to Maury Rosenbaum, who publishes the newsletter *The Diabetic Traveler* (P.O. Box 8223 RW, Stamford, CT 06905), ice actually preserves germs. He also advises always ordering carbonated water ("with gas") as carbonation adds acid and acidity kills microorganisms.

Brush your teeth using either bottled water or water you've boiled. Beware of carafes of water left on your dresser. They may well have been filled from the tap.

When all preventive measures fail, you should take some kind of antidiarrhea remedy. You'll need to consult your own doctor on this, but Dr. Peter Lodewick, writing in *The Diabetic Man,* recommends Lomotil and Imodium for diarrhea and Pepto-Bismol for nausea and cramping.

Besides taking a remedy for diarrhea, try to drink a cup of broth every hour and have bananas as your fruit exchange. This restores vital salts and potassium that are lost from your system in bouts of diarrhea. An effective folk remedy is camomile tea, known in Spanish as *té de manzanilla.*

Is it all right for me to have my ears pierced? Wear acrylic nails? Have a face-lift?

It seemed to be a good idea to group all these appearance-enhancing questions together since they have basically the same answer.

We first became aware of the ear-piercing problem when Barbara had hers pierced. She was made to sign a consent slip stating that she didn't have diabetes. Since she isn't diabetic, signing it posed no problem, but it did set her to thinking that it didn't seem fair to keep diabetics from getting their ears pierced if they wanted to. We checked with some of our experts.

Richard K. Bernstein, diabetic diabetologist of Mamaroneck, New York, was of the opinion that the restriction made sense because the vast majority of diabetics are in such poor control that it would be an infection risk for them.

Diana Guthrie, a diabetes nurse specialist, had a more positive approach: "So long as your blood sugars are normalized or near normalized, there should be no hesitation whatsoever in getting your ears pierced if the proper precautions that are taken for everybody else are taken for you."

Assuming you take care of this risk factor, you're left with only the dilemma of whether to sign the paper saying that you're *not* diabetic. Since the ear-piercing brigade is probably having you sign only to protect itself in the event of an infection, it would seem that all you're doing is denying yourself legal recourse if something should go wrong. But whether to sign is a moral question rather than a diabetic one, and we aren't the best source of the answer.

The reason we brought up the question of acrylic nails is that we know diabetics are more susceptible to nail fungus than others. Attaching these nails might therefore cause fungus to develop or spread. Diana Guthrie again set our minds at ease. She explains: "Glued-on nails do not enhance the development of fungal infections so long as careful hand-washing techniques are routinely instituted and the fungal organism is not overwhelmingly present." One of our former SugarFree employees, Melanie Epperson, who had her own nail business, echoed this sentiment. She had several diabetic clients who had acrylic nails, and not one had ever had a problem with them.

And now we get to the biggie—a face-lift. We won't debate here the advisability of cosmetic surgery (which is questionable unless the surgery is done to correct something like a cleft palate or to repair the ravages of an accident). If you do decide, for whatever personal reasons, that you would like to have a face-lift, the question is, Should your diabetes stand in your way? Again we hear good news from Diana Guthrie: "The advisability of anyone getting a face-lift or other cosmetic surgery is the same as for any surgical procedure. If someone has diabetes and it is *under control,* they probably will heal faster and better than even the nondiabetic. There should be no hesitation to do surgical procedures, so long as the service of a knowledgeable physician is available to manage the diabetes before, during, and after the procedure." Lois Jovanovic-Peterson agrees. This goes along with her philosophy that diabetics who are in control can do virtually anything they'd do if they weren't diabetic.

So the answer to all these questions (and all of life) is yes, if your diabetes is *under control.*

Is it all right to use generic drugs?

Before we answer that, we'd like you to have an understanding of what generic drugs are. We'd long been confused about them ourselves, so we asked Mike Voelker, formerly a pharmacist with SugarFree Centers, to explain them. The first thing we found out surprised us: Pharmacies actually make a greater percentage of profit on generics than on brand names, so if your pharmacist discourages you from purchasing a certain generic, he's doing it for professional reasons and not out of some sordid profit motive.

Mike further explains that generic drugs (drugs not protected by trademark) are in demand today for many valid reasons. First, insurance companies and other health-cost payment systems are encouraging their members to use generic drugs by offering people a lower copayment if they do. Second, the FDA is shortening the time period for trade-name drugs to become generic. And third, over the next three to four years, if the federal government (Medicare) phases in payments for prescription drugs (just as the state of California now does with its Medi-Cal drug program), it will probably demand that generic medications be provided whenever possible.

For the above reasons, it's safe to say that generics are here to stay. But . . . buyer, beware! Some warnings are in order. Brand-name drugs and their generic forms are not necessarily identical. Switching to a generic without proper precautions may cause serious problems. To understand the possible difficulties, you have to understand what generic drugs are and how they're made.

A generic drug has exactly the same amount of the active ingredient as the trade-name product. The active ingredient by weight, however, makes up only a fraction of the total weight of the tablet or capsule. For example, a Lanoxin 0.25 milligram tablet weighs about 1.5 milligrams, but the active ingredient (Digoxin) makes up only about 10 percent of the total weight of the tablet. The other 90 percent comprises what pharmacists call excipients—fillers, binding agents, coloring, etc. It is these extra ingredients that very often determine how much of the active drug is absorbed into the bloodstream and how quickly. In some cases more drug is absorbed and in other cases less. This difference can be critical, depending on the type of drug you're using.

With the following classes of drugs, you and your doctor and pharmacist must be extremely careful when changing to the generic form:

- cardiovascular drugs (Digoxin, Inderal, etc.)
- hormone and related drugs (Premarin)
- psychotherapeutic drugs (Thorazine, Elavil, etc.)
- anticonvulsants (Dilantin)
- oral hypoglycemics (Orinase, Diabenese, etc.)

A diabetic, for example, can switch from the trade-name Orinase to the generic tolbutamide, but you should always ask your physician first. When the switch is made, you must be very diligent about testing for hyper- or hypoglycemia so you can determine whether the generic is being absorbed in the same way as the trade-name pill. Then, once you have successfully switched, you have to make sure you are always provided with that particular brand of generic, because *generics also differ from brand to brand*. This is another complication, which means that only those in the know can protect themselves from drug overdose or underdose.

With classes of drugs not on the above list, such as antibiotics and analgesics, it is perfectly okay to switch to a generic brand without any special monitoring.

The final word on generics, then, is to go ahead and enjoy the savings they offer, but make sure that you, your physician, and your pharmacist work as a team to ensure their safe and efficacious use.

For People with Type 1 (Insulin-Dependent) Diabetes

Being on insulin is like being involved in a passionate yet turbulent marriage, one of those "can't live with; can't live without" situations.

In the case of your relationship with your insulin there are times—especially after a particularly devastating or embarrassing insulin reaction—that you feel you can't possibly live with it, no, not one minute longer. But you have no choice. You and insulin are partners, locked together inextricably forever. No divorce allowed.

Admittedly, insulin is a difficult and demanding helpmate. There's the needle and the several-times-a-day injections; the constant lookout for insulin shock; the need to have something sugary available at all times; the problem of keeping medical supplies in stock; the precise food requirements, with eating too little as big a mistake as eating too much; the necessity of stuffing some therapeutic food down for insulin's sake when you're not even hungry; the inevitable snacks between meals and at bedtime; and the inability of family, friends, and co-workers to comprehend what's going on in your rocky relationship with insulin. Then there's the expense of your marriage to insulin. No one ever had a more incorrigible spendthrift of a spouse. Living with insulin uses up big dollars that you'd rather spend on pleasures—and even sometimes need to spend on necessities.

And yet despite everything, you must love your insulin. It gives you the most precious gift of all: the gift of life itself. Before its discovery in 1921, you'd have been a goner. While it's not a cure for diabetes, as some people erroneously think it is, it's the next-best thing; in fact the *only* thing there is.

So since you're stuck (!) with insulin until they find that fabled cure that's always "just ten years away," you have to make the best of it. To help you do that, we'll now give you some insulin marital counseling in the hope that you will learn to live with your insulin happily—or at least with respect and understanding—ever after and that you will celebrate your golden and even your diamond anniversary together.

What is insulin?

Insulin, as we mentioned earlier, is the hormone that helps the body cells take up sugar from the blood. As a type 1 diabetic, you must inject insulin to replace your body's lack of the hormone. The amount to be injected every day depends on whether your body is producing none or only a small amount. If it is producing none, your injections are a substitute for your own insulin; if it is producing some, you have to augment your own insulin with injections. Your physician will determine how much insulin you need and which kinds.

Insulins are constantly being improved and redesigned to make more types available and more convenient for users. This new complexity also can mean more confusion, so it pays to learn the exact types and brands you use and their characteristics.

Basically there are two categories of insulin: fast-acting and slow-acting. The fast-acting insulins include lispro (brand name Humalog), Regular, and Semi-lente. These are used before meals to control post-meal blood sugar. Humalog begins acting in one-half to one hour and has an effective duration of only two to four hours. Regular and Semi-lente begin acting within about forty-five minutes and last four to six hours. The slow-acting insulins are divided into two types:

intermediate-acting and long-acting. Intermediate-acting insulins are Neutral Protamine Hagedorn (NPH) and Lente. These begin acting in about an hour and a half and last approximately twelve to eighteen hours. Ultralente is the only long-acting insulin. It begins to take effect in one to three hours and can last up to thirty-six hours. Most diabetics take a combination of fast-acting and intermediate- or long-acting insulins.

Injectable insulins come in bottles of ten cubic centimeters each. Fast-acting insulin is clear, and slow-acting is cloudy. Insulin is measured in units. All insulin sold in the United States is of the same concentration: U100, which means that there are one hundred units of insulin in each cubic centimeter. So a ten-cubic-centimeter bottle would contain one thousand units of insulin. If your dosage of insulin is ten units a day, then a bottle of insulin will contain one hundred doses.

Most insulins are now synthetic human insulins made in laboratories by DNA technology. Since human insulin is identical to the body's own, it does not cause antibodies or allergic reactions and is absorbed more quickly. All insulin used to be made from the pancreas of pigs and steers, but these are being phased out. Oddly enough, though, not all old-time diabetics can successfully switch to human insulin and maintain the same control they had with animal insulin. (June is one of these.) Because of this problem a minority of people both here and abroad are protesting the discontinuance of animal insulin, but at the present time the chances of persuading manufacturers to serve these people does not look particularly hopeful because of economic constraints. (Translation: Because of the small market, it doesn't pay the companies to produce it.)

Whatever insulin you use, it's a good idea when you go shopping for insulin to take the empty bottle with you and show it to the pharmacist. That way there can be no confusion. Another tip; keep a backup supply of at least one bottle in your refrigerator. Not all pharmacies stock all varieties of insulin, and you may dash out to replace your vial only to find that the pharmacy has none.

Why can't I just take my insulin in a pill?

Insulin is a protein, and if it were delivered in pill form, the stomach would digest it the way it would a hamburger; you'd get no benefit from it. Researchers are now working on encapsulating insulin in a substance that would allow it to pass through the stomach without being digested and then be released in the intestine, but they have been working on it for a long time.

Other techniques being investigated are a nasal spray and insulin patches. Keep your fingers crossed.

Once you start taking insulin, do you have to take it for the rest of your life?

If you're a type 1 diabetic, yes. Occasionally after children or young people are first diagnosed and start using insulin, there comes a honeymoon period. The disease seems to fade away, they can stop taking insulin, and their family believes a miracle has occurred and they are cured. Not so. Like all honeymoons, the diabetes honeymoon eventually comes to an end, and insulin injections must begin again. (But enjoy it while it lasts.)

Sometimes if you're a type 2, you may be on insulin only until you get your weight down.

Also, diabetics who aren't normally on insulin may have to take it when they're sick or have an infection or are pregnant. When they're well again, or the baby is delivered, they can stop.

Where and how do I inject insulin?

Insulin can be injected into the arm, abdomen, buttocks, or thigh. To make sure you stay within the proper area of each of these sites, you can order the pamphlet *Site Selection and Rotation* from Becton-Dickinson Consumer Products, One Becton Drive, Franklin Lakes, NJ 07417-1883 (1-800-237-4554).

It's very important to rotate your injections within each area, because there are differences in the speed with which insulin is absorbed, depending on where it is injected. Injection in the abdomen is fastest—30 to 50 percent faster than in other areas; next fastest are arms and legs. The usual lag time for the abdomen is 30 to 40 minutes, while in the arm or leg the time lag is usually around 40 to 50 minutes. Insulin also acts faster in places that are lean rather than fat. According to Dr. Jay S. Skyler, professor of medicine, pediatrics, and psychology at the University of Miami School of Medicine, it is preferable to inject all before-meal shots of regular insulin into the abdomen for faster action. This will help prevent post-meal blood sugar from being too high.

Humalog insulin is an exception to the preceding instructions. It can be injected anywhere and it absorbs at the same rate.

How and when do I inject insulin?

Your doctor or nurse educator will teach you the injection technique and help you practice until you feel confident, though not necessarily as relaxed about it as you'd like to. The doctor will prescribe the type or types of insulin to use and the dosage.

Standard instructions have always been to take your insulin shot one half hour before eating. (Humalog is an exception—only fifteen minutes in advance.) However, if you test your blood sugar before your meals—and you should!—it's preferable to use your test result as a guide to timing. The rationale behind this is that you can make adjustments in injection timing so the insulin's peak action will match the entry of glucose into your blood from the food you eat. Glucose starts arriving in your intestinal tract within ten minutes of eating, but insulin doesn't even begin to get going for over fifteen minutes. That's why the timing guidelines developed by Drs. David S. Schade, Mark R. Burge, and Patrick J. Boyle, of the University of New Mexico School of Medicine in Albuquerque, are so valuable. They suggest that you test your blood sugar forty-five minutes before the meal, then time your insulin injection according to your blood-sugar level. These are the Schade/ Burge/Boyle guidelines for Regular insulin (not Humalog):

BLOOD SUGAR 45 MINUTES PRIOR TO MEAL	WHEN TO TAKE YOUR INSULIN
50 mg/dl or less	after you finish the meal
50 to 70 mg/dl	just before starting the meal
70 to 120 mg/dl	15 minutes before the meal
120 to 180 mg/dl	30 minutes before the meal
Over 180 mg/dl	45 minutes before the meal

Adapted from an article in *Diabetes Forecast,* July 1993, with permission of the authors.

How can I get over my fear of the needle?

First of all, don't feel you're more cowardly than anyone else. We've never met any people who enjoyed sticking themselves with a needle. (And, in fact, we'd rather not meet any.) We have met several, though, who swore they'd never be able to do it, but when the golden moment arrived they found they could, as Lady Macbeth put it, screw their courage to the sticking place.

Most insulin-dependent diabetics who inject themselves—and many do it two or three times a day for better management—get so used to it that it's fairly routine. (We won't give you the nonsense that "it becomes like brushing your teeth.")

Sometimes people can inject themselves for years without being bothered by it. Then suddenly they begin building up dread again. If you haven't yet conquered your fear or if you find it suddenly reappearing, here's what you can do about it.

- If you have the habit of worrying about the injection and how much it's going to hurt, instead picture yourself doing it easily and without pain. Positive thinking brings about positive results.
- If you've been having someone else give you shots, start giving them yourself. Not only is this necessary in case of emergencies, but you'll reinforce your feelings of competence. You may even discover that it hurts less when you do it yourself. We tend to tense our muscles when someone else is taking a poke at us.
- Relax. Those tense muscles we just mentioned not only make the shot hurt more but can also cause bruising. (And getting bruises is not a way to make yourself fear the needle less.)
- June found that when she switched from one to three shots a day, and then later on to five, an amazing change took place: she lost all dread of the needle. This may sound ridiculous, but it's true. Our explanation is that the more often you do it, the less time you'll have to build up a wall of worry. You inject your insulin as calmly as you'd do any other daily task.

A dividend you get from mastering your insulin injections is a feeling of power, an "If I can do this, I can do anything" feeling. You'll find you become a stronger person in every way.

Now, having given you this pep talk to make you positively panting with eagerness to stick yourself with a needle, we'll deliver the news that you don't have to if you don't want to. Modern technology strikes again to make diabetes self-care easier and less traumatic.

What is an injection aide?

It's a device that takes a loaded syringe and shoots it into you so quickly that you hardly know it happened. It gives you perfect injection technique, and since you don't even see the needle in the device, it does a lot toward keeping you relaxed. Not only do these devices eliminate the fear and pain, but they can reach a lot of new injection territory and

INJECTION AIDES

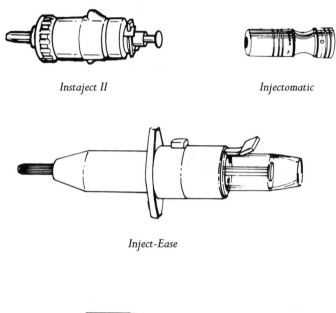

Instaject II   Injectomatic

Inject-Ease

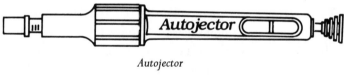

Autojector

reach it with one hand—especially important for parents of small children, for whom the statement "This hurts me more than it does you"
is often true. When a parent uses one of these devices, everybody is
happier. People with arthritis or other dexterity problems also find
these a boon. But the greatest advantage of automatic injectors is that
they facilitate the multiple injections many people need to keep their
diabetes under control and help them avoid complications.

The currently available injectors include the Injectomatic
(Kendall-Futuro), the Autojector (Ulster Scientific), the Inject-Ease
(Palco), and the Instaject II (Jordan Medical). Some are pictured here.

Most injectors can accommodate all sizes and brands of syringes. (Note: The Injectomatic is usable only with Monoject syringes, which isn't too surprising since Can-Am Care makes both.)

After the injector zaps in the needle, you press the syringe plunger to release the insulin. (With the Autojector the insulin is released automatically.)

Even with an automatic injector, though, it's true you're still using a needle, and if needles are intrinsically horrifying to you, there is yet another alternative, that is, a jet injector.

With a jet, the insulin itself becomes like a needle because it is shot in with such jetlike speed. All you feel is something like snapping your finger against your skin. You can mix insulins just as you can with needles.

But to our minds, escaping from needles is only a secondary reason for using a jet. Their greatest advantage, besides encouraging you to take more shots per day, is that they improve control, often with less insulin. When you inject with a needle, the insulin can pool at the injection site (this is called "depoting" in the trade), and the insulin is not absorbed as quickly as it should be, so it may not be there when you need it to cover a meal. Then, whammo, it's released later when you *don't* need it, and your blood sugar plummets. Jets disperse the insulin under the skin in a spray, and that explains its quicker and more uniform absorption. When insulin's action is more predictable, you have more consistent control of your blood sugar.

Jet injectors do not, of course, give ideal injections for everybody. Some people can use them and love them while others have problems. Some can get pain-free, bruise-free injections in any injection location, while others can get good shots only in the abdomen, or only in the thighs—but then that's often true of syringes as well.

Jets require a doctor's prescription. They used to have a large initial cost—in the $500-to-$700 range, but models are now as low as $399. The cost of the instrument is made up in less than three years because of savings on syringe purchases and reduced insulin requirements.

The two most experienced manufacturers and the two whose instruments June is familiar with are Medi-Ject Corporation, 1840 Berkshire Lane, Minneapolis, MN 55441 (1-800-328-3074), and Vitajet Corporation, 27075 Cabot Rd. #102, Laguna Hills, CA 92653 (1-800-848-2538).

Is the insulin-infusion pump I've heard about another way of getting off needles?

Not exactly, but it *is* a way to achieve the best possible control. That is why 59 percent of the intensive group in the DCCT were on pump therapy at least part of the time, and most of them chose to stay on it when the study ended, if they could afford to when they had to pay the costs themselves (see table on page 100).

Dr. Alan O. Marcus, writing in *Practical Diabetology* (November 1992), defined those people who are the best prospects for pump therapy or, as the physicians call it, "continuous subcutaneous insulin infusion." You are a good candidate if (1) you desire life-style flexibility, (2) you have unacceptable diabetes control, (3) you have chronic complications of diabetes, or (4) you want to become pregnant. The strongest candidates are those whose life-style is "active and variable." Physicians always stress that to be successful on a pump you must be highly motivated to use one, because pumps are not an *easier* way to good control, but a *better* way.

Pumps have been in use for almost twenty years and have become highly sophisticated marvels of technology. They are now compact and sturdy, weigh only a little over three ounces, and are battery operated and highly programmable.

You wear the pump on a belt or strapped to your leg or anywhere it's convenient. At specific intervals the pump delivers Regular insulin only. Regular insulin acts consistently, unlike intermediate and long-acting insulins, which have unpredictable absorption. The insulin travels through a slender, flexible tube and enters your body via a needle or, better still, a cannula (a tiny plastic tube) that is inserted under your skin at any normal injection site, usually the abdominal area. The needle or cannula stays in place for one to three days and then is rotated to a different spot, just as you change injection sites when using syringes and needles.

When it's time for a meal, you press a button to release the appropriate amount of regular insulin to cover the meal. Most pump wearers figure their mealtime insulin needs by testing their blood sugar and then counting the grams of carbohydrates they're going to eat.

One of the most valuable features of modern pumps is their programmability. For example, people who inject long-acting insulin often get low blood sugar in the middle of the night and then their blood sugar goes up in the very early morning (a condition known as the dawn phenomenon). The pump wearer can program the pump to deliver less insulin during the period when blood sugar is likely to be down and more insulin for the dawn blood-sugar rise.

You have to work very closely with your diabetes health care team during the period when you're finding out what your body's metabolic requirements are for insulin, the daily fluctuations of your blood sugar, and how insulin-sensitive or insulin-resistant you are in order to discover how much insulin will cover how many grams of carbohydrate for you. But after all that's worked out, you can have amazing control and amazing flexibility in your life-style and mealtimes.

The best way for you to understand what pump wearing is like is to hear it from pump wearers themselves. First, here's Pat Ockel of San Diego:

> I got my MiniMed just before I went on an African safari in June 1987. It was one of the smallest pumps available at that time and it could get wet without being harmed; it had the largest reservoir (it carried three hundred units of insulin); and it worked off three small batteries that could be found at most drugstores, even in Africa.

After I got my MiniMed pump, my husband said that my moods really smoothed out compared to when I was on shots. Also, I haven't had any bad reactions the way I used to with syringes. The strange thing is that, since I use a Sof-set instead of having a needle inserted all the time, I'm not actually aware that it's there. And it certainly makes it convenient for eating at restaurants when you just pull the pump out and take your dose right at the table.

And now here's Tom Chuchvara of Van Nuys, California:

I had been on insulin injections for nine years when low blood sugars became frequent, unpredictable, and at times life-threatening. I tested ten to twelve times a day and sometimes in the middle of the night to catch them before they happened, but I could not predict them.

I was sure the lows were due to my physically active life-style of drumming, surfing, running, and weightlifting. I finally decided that a choice had to be made: either reduce the physical activity or find a program compatible with it. That's when I discovered the Disetronic H-Tron V100 insulin pump. This pump provides a feature that allows the user to adjust the rate at which insulin is pumped in order to match the level of physical activity at any given time.

The Disetronic has been part of my new program for over a year now. It allows me to manage my diabetes in accordance with my diet and the type of physical activity I choose, including surfing. My diabetes management has improved tremendously and I am now under good control. High and low blood sugars are extremely rare, and I am free to live as I want to.

For further information on pumps, write or call Disetronic Medical Systems, Inc., 5201 East River Road, Ste. 312, Minneapolis, MN 55421-1014 (1-800-688-4578) or MiniMed Technologies, Inc., 12744 San Fernando Rd., Sylmar, CA 91342 (1-800-933-3322).

What if I forget to take my insulin injection?

At least you'll know you're not obsessed with your disease. But if this happens more than once in a great while, you'll need to devise some kind of reminder system, like a nagging husband, wife, or parent. If you have small children, you can give them a penny each time you take the shot. (They'll never forget, but don't let them con you into taking your shot twice.) When it does dawn on you that you forgot your shot, take your blood sugar and see what's happening. Call your doctor, who can probably help you decide how much insulin to take, if any. Much depends on what kind of insulin you take and how many shots a day you take, so general advice is of no help.

Sometimes the problem is even worse. It's remembering whether or not you took the insulin. Then you have to worry about getting a double dose or no dose at all. If you're at a total loss and can't figure out whether you did or didn't, the safer course is not to take a shot. Think how tough it would be and how much time it would take to eat all the extra food the double injection would require, not to mention the weight it would put on. There's no doubt that a good memory is a help to a diabetic.

When I'm sick and can't eat—do I stop taking insulin?

That's a good question, as politicians being interviewed by reporters like to say. The answer is no, no, a thousand times no. If you have severe nausea and vomiting and can't keep anything down, you can sometimes reduce your normal daily insulin dose by one-half or two-thirds (if your blood sugars are normal). But more often when you're sick, your blood sugar goes up and you need more insulin, not less. (Illness makes insulin less effective.) Sometimes your doctor (keep in touch when you're sick) will prescribe additional shots of fast-acting insulin before each meal.

For sick days when you can't eat solid food, the usual recommendation is to sip ginger ale (to control nausea and to satisfy your insulin) and to drink clear broth or fruit juices every hour.

Whenever you're sick, especially with the flu, a cold, an injury, or an infection, you have to watch your diabetes more closely. Take your blood sugar every few hours. If it's over 240, check your urine for ketones. If ketones appear, call your doctor immediately. Blood-sugar levels can go very high during illness, and your doctor can help you bring them down safely. But don't just sit there—or lie there—and do nothing. This is not a situation you can safely ignore.

Do insulin syringes and needles require a prescription?

This one's a real puzzler. The answer is that they do and they don't. In California, for example, most pharmacists require only the diabetic's signature, not the doctor's. Some states, however, insist on a doctor's prescription. The laws vary from state to state, and the interpretation of the laws varies from pharmacy to pharmacy.

We've never tried purchasing this equipment out of state or overseas, but June always carries a doctor's prescription in case the occasion should ever arise.

Do I need to clean the skin with alcohol before I inject?

We hate to advocate unhygienic practices, but we also hate for you to get all agitated and upset if you don't have any alcohol or an alcohol swab along when you need to take a shot.

For what it's worth, June never cleans the injection site with alcohol—unless, of course, she hasn't been able to bathe on a daily basis. One doctor told us there was a British study in which they gave five thousand injections using alcohol and five thousand without. There were only five infections in the whole lot, and all those were in cases where alcohol had been used! (The doctor laughed and said maybe the alcohol irritated the bacteria and stirred them into action.)

How do I take care of my bottles of insulin?

Bottles is the correct word, because you should have more than one on hand. The backup supply should be kept in the refrigerator (not in the coldest part, where it might freeze, and certainly not in the freezer compartment). The vial you're using (or vials, if you use more than one kind) can stay at room temperature, providing it is not over 86 degrees Fahrenheit. Insulin manufacturers usually recommend refrigeration between shots, but cold insulin causes more pain when injected and does not absorb as well. Insulin usually remains stable for much more than a month, even though manufacturers tell you to discard open vials after a month. It ordinarily is stable for at least three months without refrigeration. Always write the date you opened it on the bottle so you'll know where you are timewise with it.

You should, by the way, always watch the expiration date on your insulin. If you use it after that date, it may not be as effective. For that reason, you can't stock up on huge quantities of insulin when you find it on sale. That's not a good idea anyway, as you might change insulins.

It's perfectly okay to carry your insulin in your purse or pocket (in a protective case of some kind) when you're not going to be taking your injection at home. Insulin is pretty hardy stuff. You just have to be careful not to freeze it or expose it to high temperatures (above 100 degrees Fahrenheit), or to jiggle it around too much.

When traveling you don't have to worry about keeping your insulin refrigerated, but you do have to worry about where to keep it. In airplanes, don't put your insulin in the luggage you check. Keep it in your pocket, purse, or hand luggage, both because the cargo hold may be too cold and because your luggage may get lost along the way. If you're traveling by automobile, don't leave your insulin in a closed car in the hot sun because the temperature can rise to damaging heights.

Many people wisely buy an insulated carrying case for insulin, especially if they're planning a trip to an extremely hot or cold climate. When traveling by plane you should always keep your insulin in one of these insulated cases. This is especially true in long-distance flights where we've heard they often do what's known in the airline biz as "coshing"—turning up the cabin temperature to make the passengers drowsy and undemanding. June once had her whole supply of (uninsulated) insulin ruined on a flight from Los Angeles to Rome. She couldn't buy the insulin she uses in Italy, so she was semi-out-of-control the whole trip. She learned her lesson the hard way, and now she gives it the care it deserves in an insulated case.

Each year the October issue of *Diabetes Forecast* has a "Buyer's Guide to Diabetes Products," which lists all carrying cases available. In 1997 it included eleven different cases with cold packs, plus eight without, that protect your insulin when you're carrying it around with you. These are described and special features given. It's almost essential to have some form of carrying case for travel. Cases can often be ordered by mail order. Just watch the advertisements.

What causes those lumps that I sometimes get after a shot?

It could be that you've injected too frequently in the same place or that you're allergic to the kind of insulin you're using—or both. Try to be more conscientious about rotating the injection site. If the lumps continue to appear, tell your doctor, who may change the type of insulin you're using.

Some people get skin indentations or depressions instead of lumps. These are caused by losing fat wherever you inject insulin (fat atrophy). The correction for both problems, if you aren't on human insulin now, is often to change to human.

Can I get along on one shot of intermediate-acting insulin a day?

Almost definitely not. The therapeutic life of human NPH (the length of time it controls blood sugar) is only twelve to fourteen hours. The other intermediate-acting insulin, Lente, controls for only fourteen to sixteen hours. You can see that using only one shot of either of these insulins would leave you uncovered for a lot of time during a twenty-four-hour period. Not only that, but taking it in one shot would mean that the insulin would peak once, possibly at a time when you very likely wouldn't have planned to have your main meal. You'd have to feed your insulin when it demanded it and then not be able to eat when you (and everyone else) wanted to. So not only is one shot bad therapy, it makes for a rigid and unpleasant life.

Dr. Lois Jovanovic-Peterson does admit that people who still have some pancreatic function, mostly type 2's, can get along on only one shot of NPH. If you always have normal fasting blood sugars on the one-shot-a-day plan, you are among the few lucky ones who can do it. Dr. Jovanovic-Peterson emphasizes, though, that the vast majority of type 1 diabetics who have no pancreatic function can't possibly have good control with one shot of NPH a day—no matter how much they'd love to do it.

You keep talking about taking all those injections to keep blood sugar normal. How do I handle it when I'm out at restaurants?

It's not all that difficult, thanks to the many helpful devices the diabeticization of America has produced.

You can load your syringe at home and carry it in a Wright's Pre-filled Syringe Case, which is made of polypropylene and looks like a fountain pen. You can order it from the manufacturer, LLW Enterprises, P.O. Box 591353, Houston, TX 77259-1353 (281-480-1506); the cost is $16.95 for two. With this case, it's quick and easy to take your shot in the restaurant restroom or even in the car prior to entering the restaurant, even if the lighting isn't bright enough for measuring your dosage.

Another system that's particularly handy for injecting away from home is the portable preloaded insulin pen. An example is the Novo Pen 1.5. You load it with a cartridge of Novolin regular, NPH, or 70/30 (70 percent NPH, 30 percent regular). Each cartridge contains 150 units of insulin. You can dial in the number of units you want to take (from 1 to 40 in 1-unit increments) and shoot it in. You change the disposable needle at the end of the pen after each shot.

The latest thing for people who take 70/30 insulin is the Novolin 70/30 Prefilled, a disposable syringe prefilled with 150 units of Novolin 70/30 human insulin. You use it with the disposable needles of the NovolinPen. It lasts from three to five days, depending on your dosage.

Becton-Dickinson offers the B-D Pen and the B-D Pen Mini, as well as their new Ultra-Fine needles in both standard and short lengths. The Mini, a 15-unit pen, is distinctive in that it measures in one-half-unit increments. The Mini is at present available only by mail order (call 1-800-400-7367). The current price is $39.50, including shipping and handling. Both these pens use Lilly or Novo Nordisk insulin cartridges.

How do I adjust my insulin when I fly and change time zones?

That depends strictly on your insulin schedule, what kind of insulin you take, and how many shots a day you require. And there's more than one method for calculating the adjustments.

To give you a basic understanding of the problem, remember that time change occurs only when you fly east or west, not north or south.

Flying from west to east, your day is shortened. Flying from east to west, it is lengthened. So when flying east, you lower your dosage; when flying west, you increase it. *But* if the change is not more than four hours, you don't need to take any special action. Likewise, if your total insulin dose is small—only ten or fifteen units—you can probably get by without any change.

If you monitor your blood sugar frequently, you can stay out of trouble and in control, no matter what. Knowing how to adjust insulin according to blood sugar and giving yourself supplements of Regular or Humalog insulin makes the whole thing easy. Otherwise, discuss your insulin program well ahead of the trip with your physician or nurse educator.

Airborne-injection tip: When you take an insulin injection in a plane, do not inject air into the bottle. If you do, because of the difference in air pressure the plunger will fight you and make it difficult to measure accurately.

Is it all right to have low blood sugar?

No. Low blood sugar—or insulin reaction, as low blood sugar is often called—can be very hazardous for a diabetic because you become irritable, befuddled, uncoordinated, and, in extreme cases, unconscious. Automobile accidents are not the only possible danger. One of our friends fell in his swimming pool when he blacked out during an insulin reaction and was lucky enough to be awakened by the water and make it to the side and climb out. Maybe you read the story of Candy Sangster, who became unconscious during a weekend at home alone. She was saved by her dog, Jet, who went outside and barked until the neighbors decided to dial 911. Jet, a six-year-old Doberman, was named the Ken-L-Ration Dog Hero of the Year in 1986 for his dramatic life-saving exploit. So if you don't own a hero dog, don't be lax about hypoglycemia.

The most logical way to check to see if you're having an insulin reaction is to take your blood sugar. You should also learn to recognize the characteristic physical and/or mental changes that take place. The difficulty is not only that these are very diverse, individualized, and vary from occasion to occasion but that many people fail to notice them. Psychologist Daniel J. Cox, Ph.D., in a study published in *Diabetes Care* (February 1993) found that in his group only 50 percent of the lows were recognized. He also found out that the most frequently recognized symptoms were trembling, difficulty concentrating, confusion, and pounding heart. Notice that half of these are mental rather than physical.

A serious problem that has surfaced recently is one called "hypoglycemic unawareness" or more descriptively "hypoglycemia without warning." Robert S. Dinsmoor, in an article in *Diabetes Self-Management* (March/April 1993), explains that in the DCCT study this happened with almost half the people with longstanding diabetes (fifteen to twenty years). Intensive insulin therapy seems to accentuate the problem, as does neuropathy.

The physiological explanation for unawareness, according to Dinsmoor, is that people with diabetes lose the natural protections that keep blood sugar normal. These are the release of glucagon, which raises blood sugar, and epinephrine (also called adrenaline), which tells you with such symptoms as shaking and perspiring that it's down. Until something better comes along, the main solution is to monitor your blood sugar more frequently and *always* have glucose tablets available.

The best solution to this dilemma is to work harder to normalize your blood sugar, because your body has simply gotten used to low blood sugars. June, who for years had frequent lows in an extreme effort not to have highs, found out that when she switched to the low carbohydrate diet and established a pattern of staying constantly within a range of 70 to 120, after about two months she totally regained her symptoms of hypoglycemia, even becoming aware when she had only dropped to 60. For too many years, even at a level of 40 she would have no idea she was low.

Why do I sometimes feel as if I'm having an insulin reaction when my blood sugar is normal?

It could be that physical or psychological factors unrelated to your diabetes are making you feel strange. But we have talked to several diabetics who maintain that they feel better with high blood sugar and that when it's normal they feel as if they're hypoglycemic.

Some of those who experience this phenomenon have been running around for quite a while with high blood sugar, either because they weren't testing their blood sugar and didn't realize how high it was or because they'd just been sloppy in their diabetes care. You know the song "I've Been Down So Long It Feels Like Up to Me"? Well, these diabetics have been up so long it feels like normal to them. Consequently, when they start bringing their blood sugar down to where it should be, they feel unnatural. It's almost like coming off a drug.

But if you stick to it and keep your blood sugar in the normal range, before long you'll feel right only when your blood sugar's right.

What do I do for an insulin reaction?

You eat or drink something sweet that will bring your blood sugar up fast. (This always confuses nondiabetics, who are convinced that diabetics can *never* have anything sugary and resist giving them what they need.) Most lists of what to eat for insulin reactions have been the same for years—and still are. They include a half glass of orange juice, sugar cubes, three or four Life Savers, a half cup of Coke or Pepsi, two tablespoons of raisins, etc. We've never understood how anyone could conceive of some of these items as handy to carry in your purse or pocket at all times. And we particularly don't fathom the magic of orange juice. It's actually low on the Carbohydrate Glycemic Index (see page 46).

What you need in a low-blood-sugar emergency—and it should be treated as an emergency—is something quick and easy, good-tasting, and predictable. That's why we favor glucose tablets.

Some of the more convenient ones are Can-Am's Dex4's, Dextrotabs, and B-D Glucose Tablets. All come in different flavors except B-D (orange only). Dex4's have 4 grams of glucose per tablet, Dextrotabs have 1.6 grams, and B-Ds have 5 grams. Dex4's will raise the blood sugar of a person weighing 120 to 150 pounds by approximately fifteen milligrams per deciliter; Dextrotabs will raise it by approximately eight milligrams per deciliter; and B-Ds by approximately twenty-five milligrams per deciliter.

Most glucose tablets are available in pharmacies, and such retailers as Walgreens, Kmart, etc., have a store brand. Dextrotabs are harder to find but can be ordered from the manufacturer; the price is $19.44 for a jar of three hundred. (Call Cramer Products in Garner, KS 66030: 913-856-7511.)

The best way to find out exactly how much each of these tablets will raise *your* blood sugar is to test them on yourself. (Wait until your blood sugar is 100 or below; then eat one and retest in fifteen minutes.) If you know how many to eat for an insulin reaction, you won't make the classic mistake of overcompensating and sending yourself from 50 to 250. (This is called anxiety eating, and that term describes the phenomenon perfectly.)

If you get to the point where you are too far gone to chew but are conscious and able to swallow, the suggested treatment is one of the jels that can be absorbed in the mouth. These are Glutose (in a plastic container), Insta-Glucose (in a squeeze tube), and Monoject Insulin Reaction Gel (foil-wrapped pouch). A less expensive way to go is to pick up a few tubes of cake decorating icing in any supermarket.

Our final word: If you take insulin, live like a boy scout. Be prepared.

I've been told I should keep a supply of glucagon on hand. What is glucagon, and how is it used?

Glucagon is a hormone that's injected in the same way as insulin, only it has the opposite effect. It raises blood sugar. It's used to resuscitate diabetics who are unconscious because of low blood sugar.

Even if you never use it, glucagon is a nice security blanket. Just be sure whoever might be giving you an injection of glucagon knows where you keep it and how to administer it. And caution your family members or friends that if you're in insulin shock and unconscious, they should inject glucagon rather than trying to force liquid or food down your throat. An unconscious person cannot swallow and may choke to death.

Glucagon is available by prescription only. (This has never made sense to us, since insulin *isn't* a prescription medication and it's essential to have a supply of glucagon on hand if you take insulin.) It comes in the form of a Glucagon Emergency Kit made by Eli Lilly. A syringe is supplied and already filled with diluting solution that you mix with the powder. Many pharmacies do not regularly carry glucagon. When you find one that does or will order it for you, check the expiration date of the glucagon; it should be about two years in advance. Prices can be very high, so comparison shop.

I'm afraid of having an insulin reaction when I'm asleep and never waking up. Can this happen?

This is so rare that we've heard of it happening only twice. One time it was a diabetic who went to bed drunk and wound up literally dead drunk. What happened was the alcohol suppressed the body's method of spontaneous recovery. Normally, the liver converts some of its stored starch to glucose, and that saves you. The moral of this story is to always go to bed sober.

The other instance was reported to us by the sister of a young man who died. She said he was so obsessively compulsive about never having a slightly elevated blood sugar that he always played it too close. One night he went to bed and didn't wake up. His sister found his blood-sugar record book and discovered that his before-bed blood sugar was 70. Obviously, he needed a snack before bed and either didn't have one or had too little. The moral of this story is not to be a fanatic about your blood-sugar control.

Many people wake up and feel restless when they have low blood sugar in the middle of the night. In this case, take your blood sugar and if it's low, eat glucose tablets and/or drink milk. (We hope you keep your meter at your bedside.) If you're experiencing more insulin reactions than usual, set your alarm for 2 A.M. and do a test. Your regimen may need changing. Have a snack before bed if your blood sugar is less than 120–150 or speak with your doctor about altering your evening long-range insulin dose. With proper programming, a pump can easily solve this problem.

Another more recent strategy is to use Humalog insulin before dinner; since it only lasts three or four hours, it may be out of your system even before you go to sleep and cannot possibly cause a low-blood-sugar episode. Another new antidote to nighttime blood-sugar anxiety is to consume one of the new slow-acting carbohydrate bars designed especially to prevent nighttime hypoglycemia. The basis of these bars is cornstarch. Cornstarch also can be stirred into yoghurt or peanut butter for children's bedtime snacks so they will release sugar over a longer period of time. Currently the popular brands of slow-releasing bars are NiteBite (fifteen grams of carbohydrate and eight grams of protein) and Gluc-O-Bar (twenty grams of carbohydrate, eight grams of protein).

What is diabetic coma?

A diabetic coma occurs when your blood sugar is extremely high—perhaps over 1,000. You have diabetic ketoacidosis. Your sodium-bicarbonate and carbon-dioxide levels are low. You are dehydrated.

Oddly enough, you don't have to be unconscious to be in diabetic coma. Only 15 percent of those in diabetic coma are.

To define it more bluntly, diabetic coma is what out-of-control diabetics die of. Death from diabetic coma has been totally preventable since the discovery of insulin in 1921.

To avoid getting yourself into this dangerous state:

- Do your best to always keep your diabetes under control.
- Never neglect testing your blood sugar. If it's high, test for ketones, too. If there are ketones, call your doctor.
- If you are insulin-dependent, never neglect taking your injection.
- Whenever you are ill, check with your doctor to see if you need to take more insulin.

Diabetic coma approaches slowly. The symptoms are thirst, frequent urination, fever, drowsiness, rapid breathing, vomiting or nausea, and finally unconsciousness. The treatment for ketoacidosis is fast-acting insulin.

Can I get a driver's license if I take insulin?

Definitely yes. We don't know the regulations in all states, because they're all somewhat different, but we do know that the California Department of Motor Vehicles has liberal rules. Diabetics don't even have to reveal that they have diabetes unless they're subject to periods of unconsciousness.

Is it all right to drive a car alone on long trips?

Of course. You must, however, always carefully monitor your blood sugar. On *any* trip, short or long, never start out before checking your blood sugar and making sure it is normal or somewhat above normal. This should be a strict, no-exceptions-made personal law. We've heard of too many tragedies involving people with diabetes not to be fervent advocates of this policy. This is one of June's most inflexible rules, and she was lucky enough to learn it through other people's experience. Driving is dangerous enough without augmenting the risk with a fuzzy mind and an ill-coordinated body.

It goes without saying that you should have glucose tablets and snacks in the car with you. If you're on a long trip, stop at regular intervals (say, every hour) and test your blood sugar. Then you can snack enough to avoid low blood sugar. And if you take NPH or any other intermediate or long-acting insulin that programs you into certain eating hours, you should stop and eat when mealtime strikes. If you know there's a dearth of restaurants on the route or you're particular about what you eat, it's better to take along a picnic meal than to risk having to delay your meal or stoke up on snacks.

Is it okay to exercise alone if you take insulin?

It's always better to have a companion for safety's sake, as well as for company. You especially shouldn't do anything potentially hazardous like skiing or swimming alone.

Still, there isn't always somebody around, and a diabetic does always need exercise. There's no reason you can't take a walk or jog or ride your bicycle or play a round of golf by yourself. Just be sure you never leave the house without glucose tablets and enough snacks to see you through. *Enough* is the word here. Take along a lot more than you think you would possibly need. Then you'll never have to curtail your fun. Choose snacks that are good and, preferably, good for you, such as small packages of raisins or dried prunes, fruit leathers, trail mix, peanut butter and crackers, and the like.

Or for something more compact, use one of the new bars that provide carbohydrate and protein. PowerBars contain forty-five grams of carbohydrate and ten grams of protein; a Balance bar has twenty grams of carbohydrate and fifteen grams of protein; Clif bars have forty-five grams of carbohydrate and ten grams of protein. Many sports people also find it convenient to use the slow-acting carbohydrate bars originally designed to prevent nighttime hypoglycemia (see page 147) because these act as a kind of preventive basal carbohydrate supply for peace of mind.

For People with Type 2
(Non-Insulin-Dependent) Diabetes

If you find type 2 diabetes confusing and hard to understand, you're not alone. The general public doesn't understand it at all. What they think of when they hear the word "diabetes" is type 1, the kind in which you have to "stick yourself with a needle." They think this even though type 2's like you are in the vast majority—around 90 percent—of all people with diabetes. Many of them also erroneously think you got diabetes from eating too many sweets. The old "shame-on-you" factor kicks in.

Sad to say, there are also some health professionals who don't understand type 2 diabetes very well either. Some even go so far as to consider type 2 diabetes your fault. "If you weren't so overweight," they say judgmentally, "you wouldn't have diabetes." Here's another "shame-on-you" factor that's as wrong as it is cruel. (If you ever hear anything like this from a health professional, run, do not walk, out the door and never come back.)

And to make a personal confession for which we now hope to gain absolution, we, too, until recently totally misunderstood the true nature of type 2 diabetes. We considered it "a kind of life-style disease" and even perpetuated the erroneous theory that "with most type 2 diabetics, diabetes is a symptom; the real disease is overweight." But in 1992 we became enlightened. We decided to write a book for type 2's whom we had finally come to consider the "neglected majority." Our collab-orator and the person who set us straight once and for all was Virginia Valentine, R.N., C.D.E., and herself a not-thin type 2. Writing the book *Diabetes Type II and What to Do* was the educational process by which we learned what a complex and frustrating form of diabetes this is. Now we can pass our newfound knowledge on to you.

As we mentioned earlier, you were genetically programmed for this disease. It's extremely hereditary, much more so than type 1. If one twin gets type 1 diabetes, it ain't necessarily so that the other will, too. If a twin gets type 2, though, the diagnosis of the other twin is almost invariably not far behind. In fact, we bet that if you climb around your family tree, you'll find you have a type 2 diabetic up there somewhere—maybe on your own branch. This genetic programming for type 2 makes your cells unreceptive to insulin. (Remember, insulin is like a key that unlocks the cells to let the glucose in to fuel the body.)

You were also genetically programmed to be overweight. You have thrifty genes that cause you to store calories more easily than those around you, even when you eat less than they do. This would make you a great survivor during a famine period or in a prison camp where they feed you a starvation diet, but it compounds your problem with your genetic disposition toward insulin resistance, since extra weight makes you even more resistant.

If you're a woman, you have another built-in weight-magnet. Women have a slower metabolism than men. If a man and a woman of the same general build eat the same number of calories and do the same amount of exercise, the woman is likely to put on weight while the man stays the same or even loses. This is nature's way of protecting pregnant women and their babies-to-be during times of low food sup-ply. Nature can't seem to understand that you don't need this protec-tion when you're neither pregnant nor starving. But at any rate, this slower metabolism is what helps make type 2 diabetes more common in women than men.

Another general misconception is that all diabetics lack insulin. Again, that's only true for type 1's. You probably have plenty of insulin, maybe even an excess amount. Your cells are just resistant to it or don't have enough receptors or both. Your poor old pancreas keeps pumping out more insulin in a valiant effort to get those cells to open up and let the insulin and glucose do their thing. But it doesn't work. All that happens is that the insulin, which is a great fat-producing and storing hormone, makes you feel hungry all the time, so you eat more and put on more weight, and this makes your cells even more resistant, and more and more sugar (glucose) is floating around your bloodstream. Since it can't get into the cells, your body stores a lot of this sugar as fat. This makes you even more insulin-resistant.

The last straw is that the liver, whose job it is to release glucose when it's needed by the body, gets the impression that it's time to do its job because, since no glucose is getting into the cells, it figures there must be no glucose in the bloodstream. (Obviously, the liver doesn't understand type 2 diabetes very well either!) At any rate, the liver ("I'm just doing my job") pours forth glucose, and your blood sugar goes ever higher. It goes so high that it is finally in the diabetic range. Ergo, you have type 2 diabetes.

From all this, you can see it's not your fault that you have diabetes. As Virginia Valentine says loud and clear in *Diabetes Type II and What to Do,* "Diabetes is not a character flaw!"

What does it mean to be told you're a "borderline" diabetic?

It means the person who told you that has a very loose grasp on what diabetes is all about. There is no such thing as borderline diabetes. The term has been totally outmoded since 1979. In fact, it never should have been used in the first place. The ADA in 1997 set new standards for the diagnosis of diabetes. If you have a fasting blood-sugar level of over 126, you can consider yourself diabetic. No borderline about it.

We might mention here that according to these new guidelines for the diagnosis and classification of diabetes, certain people should be checked for diabetes more often than every three years after the age of forty-five, which is the usual recommendation. See if you fall into any of these groups:

- are obese (20 percent or more above ideal body weight)
- have a first-degree relative with diabetes
- are a member of a high-risk ethnic group (African American, Hispanic, Native American, Asian)
- have delivered a baby weighing more than nine pounds or were diagnosed with gestational diabetes
- are hypertensive (blood pressure at or above 140/90)
- have an HDL cholesterol level (the "good" cholesterol) of 35 mg/dl or lower and/or a triglyceride level of 250 mg/dl or higher

I've heard that type 2 diabetes isn't as serious as type 1 diabetes. Is this true?

It's about as true as saying that if you forget about diabetes it will go away. We wish it were true, because then instead of sixteen million diabetics in the United States there would be only one million. And we wish it were true for your sake, if you are a type 2, because that would mean you could relax and put your condition in the same category as a food allergy or a case of eczema.

No, it's not true. Type 2 diabetes is just as serious as type 1, and, like type 1, it will, if ignored or neglected, eventually cause health problems that are just as severe. The only difference is that the pattern of the development of these problems and their types may be somewhat different. Uncontrolled type 2 diabetes leads most often to heart disease, strokes, high blood pressure, and foot problems, while uncontrolled type 1 diabetes is more likely to create eye, kidney, and nerve damage (in scientific terms, retinopathy, nephropathy, and neuropathy, respectively). Of course, type 2's can develop any of those complications also. In fact, Priscilla Hollander, M.D., writing in *Learning to Live Well with Diabetes,* says, "Neuropathy seems to appear earlier in people with type 2 diabetes. In fact, it may be the first sign that a person has type 2 diabetes."

A more positive piece of information is that these threats to your health do not develop fast. It takes eight or ten or even fifteen years for the body gradually to succumb to them. You do have to consider, however, that if you had high blood sugar several years before you were diagnosed diabetic, some damage could have been done before you were aware of your diabetes. This would explain why the development of neuropathy might be the first clue to your doctor that you have developed diabetes. As with many other diseases, the sooner you discover you have diabetes, the better off you are, because you can start normalizing your blood sugar and thereby prevent or reverse complications.

If you put two and two together you'll see that the leading complications of type 2 diabetes are the same as those problems that tend to develop as you move into your more advanced years: heart disease, strokes, and high blood pressure. The most significant of these is high blood pressure. It's an astounding fact that between 45 and 50 percent of type 2's—regardless of their ethnic background or other risk factors—also have high blood pressure. The synergetic effect of type 2 diabetes and aging can be worsened even more if your life-style has been and continues to be unhealthy (very little exercise, high-fat diet, smoking, etc.) and your family has a history of these diseases. All the more reason to play it safe and follow the life-style of the growing numbers of active, health-conscious seniors we now have in this country. And diabetes will show you the way.

Can children have type 2 diabetes?

Yes, they can. It's called MODY (maturity-onset diabetes of the young; see page 10). It occurs infrequently, and, according to *The Johns Hopkins*

Guide to Diabetes, it "is seen more often in African-Americans and is now known to be due to a specific genetic defect which is unrelated to type 1 diabetes." Here's the word on it from two authorities: Richard Guthrie, M.D., co-director of the Mid-America Diabetes Associates Program and director of the Diabetes Treatment Center at St. Joseph's Medical Center in Wichita, and Diana Guthrie, R.N., Ph.D., professor at the University of Kansas School of Medicine in Wichita.

> Overweight children with high blood-sugar levels are brought to our attention by referral from other physicians or parents who are concerned about the weight problem in the child. When we do a glucose-tolerance test on them, we also analyze for insulin values. These particular children, who usually have high glucose levels as well as high insulin values, return to normal laboratory values in most cases once weight loss has been achieved. We have not followed them to find out about complications, but we have seen some children in this descriptive category become type 2 diabetics. The main treatment, of course, is increasing the activity level with the ultimate goal of decreasing the weight. Usually, the children are not on restricted caloric intake, but we work very strongly with maintaining the caloric intake and increasing the activity level.

Since I don't take insulin, do I have to do all that blood-sugar testing?

Absolutely. All diabetics who want to keep normal blood-sugar levels, and that should be your goal, have to test their blood sugar to assure themselves that they are staying on track. No way out. Well, there is an illusory way out. You may have been put on old-fashioned urine-sugar testing instead of blood-sugar testing and led to believe that if there is no sugar in your urine, your blood sugar is okay. Supposedly, no sugar in the urine means you are staying under 180—the normal renal threshold, as it is called. It is the normal level at which sugar moves into the urine in a desperate attempt to keep you out of what Dr. Peter Forsham calls "glucotoxicity" (sugars high enough to poison your system).

But this is the rub: Since most people are older when diagnosed and the renal threshold goes up with age, finding no sugar in your urine may simply mean that your renal threshold has edged up; your blood sugar might still be dangerously high. This is common with older type 2's who may have been introduced to urine testing years ago when it was the only test you could take.

For example, we talked to the daughter of a diabetic woman who, according to her daughter, "*loves* to eat, especially at big family gatherings." The mother would take her urine test, it would show that she wasn't spilling sugar, and so, presuming her blood sugar to be normal, she'd sit down happily and, as her daughter put it, "have a feast."

The woman wound up in the hospital with dangerous ketoacidosis. She'd been running extremely high blood sugar, but it had never shown up in her urine because of her high renal threshold.

This woman is now testing her blood sugar regularly at home. She doesn't have many feasts these days, but she's going to be around for a lot more normal meals than she would have been had she continued to dwell in a diabetes fool's paradise with her urine tests.

Another insidious aspect about being casual with your self-care and testing is that if you run around too long with elevated blood sugar, those diabetes complications we're always talking about can start slowly and quietly developing. You may never even know what is going on until the damage is done. We're not fearmongers, and we don't like to threaten you with the problems diabetics are heir to, but in our experience many non-insulin-dependent diabetics don't get the point about the seriousness of diabetes the way insulin takers do.

Remember that even if you don't take insulin, you have to be as careful as if you did. Actually, type 2's are the most likely candidates for arrival at the hospital with diabetes-related complications or, as Professor Diana Guthrie warns, "to have to have part of a leg removed," because they're the ones most likely to ignore their diabetes until it screams for attention.

*My doctor has prescribed pills to help me control my
blood-sugar levels. What are these, and are they safe?*

They are what the doctors call oral hypoglycemic agents (OHAs).
Translation: They are pills that help lower blood sugar in some type 2
diabetics. They are not oral insulin, as some people think. (Insulin cannot effectively be taken orally, as it is a protein and would be digested.)

The original OHAs all belong to one class, the sulfonylureas.
They have been used for over forty years. Sulfonylureas encourage the
pancreas to make more insulin, but when the pancreas becomes incapable of doing so, as often happens with time, the sufonylureas are no
longer effective.

The table below shows the entire choice of sulfonylurea drugs
now available.

ORAL HYPOGLYCEMICS

GENERIC NAME	TRADE NAME	AVAILABLE DOSAGE STRENGTHS, TABLETS (MG)	MAXIMUM DOSAGE (GM/DAY)	DURATION ACTION (HOURS)
FIRST GENERATION				
Tolbutamide	Orinase	250–500	2.0–3.0	6–12
Chlorpropamide	Diabinese	100–250	0.5	up to 600
Acetohexamide	Dymelor	250–500	1.5	12–24
Tolazamide	Tolinase	100–250–500	1.5	10–16
SECOND GENERATION				
Glyburide	Micronase®	1.25–2.5 to 5	20 mg	18–30
Glyburide	Diabeta®	1.25–2.5 to 5	20 mg	18–30
Glipizide	Glucotrol®	5 to 10	40 mg	14–20
Glimepiride	Amaryl	4	8 mg	24

The first generation of sulfonylureas (known generically as tolbu-tamide, chlorpropamide acetohexamide, and tolazamide) carry an FDA warning about their causing an increased risk of heart attack (just what you don't need). The second generation of oral hypoglycemics (gener-ically called glyburide and glipizide), which came into use in the United States in 1984, are much more potent and are considered safer in that they cause fewer side effects because the dosage is smaller and they do not interact with other drugs.

If you fail on the sulfonylureas, there is now a choice of three more OHAs, one of which may work for you. Here are the latest se-lections:

1. Glucophage (metformin) is as effective as sulfonylureas but without the risk of hypoglycemia; it lowers blood glucose by decreasing in-sulin resistance and helps decrease or stabilize body weight. It's con-traindicated for people with renal insufficiency or impairment because it causes lactic acidosis (a life-threatening complication).

2. Acarbose (precose) works in a very different way from any of the other drugs. It slows the absorption of carbohydrates in the intestine and therefore limits the post-meal blood-sugar surge. Flatulence is a common side effect.

3. Rezulin (troglitazone) has two main effects. It increases the absorp-tion of glucose by the muscles and reduces the glucose output of the liver. It does not cause weight gain or hypoglycemia. It's mainly being used for type 2's who do not have good control in spite of taking in-sulin. There is a rare but dangerous liver problem associated with Rezulin's use. In fact, in December 1997 it was pulled off the mar-ket in Great Britain, but the FDA announced at that time that it con-tinued "to find the benefits outweigh the risks if doctors follow the liver-testing recommendations."

More new drugs are being developed. For instance, Novo Nordisk's new type 2 drug became available in April of 1998. Its brand name is Prandin. It is taken about fifteen minutes before each meal and boosts insulin production at the ideal time—just when mealtime blood glucose surges.

Oral-drug therapy is a next-to-the-last-resort treatment for type 2 diabetes. The first line of defense is diet and exercise. Then if blood sugars do not retreat, the person is a candidate for some kind of pill. If pills alone don't cause improvement, you can take advantage of a new technique being tried: combining pills with one shot of insulin a day, usually a small amount of intermediate-acting NPH at bedtime. The disadvantage here is that the insulin may increase obesity.

Obviously, if you fail on the pills the next step is insulin.

Insulin?! I thought I had non-insulin-dependent diabetes. Why are we talking about insulin?

A lot of people believe that type 2's never have to take insulin unless they take it temporarily when they're ill or have surgery or some other stress to the body. Unfortunately, a lot of people are wrong. The truth, according to our type 2 guru, Virginia Valentine, is that "as many as 25 to 50 percent of type 2's will eventually be using insulin to manage their diabetes."

The first step in type 2 management is keeping your blood sugar in control, using diet and exercise. If that works, fine. You have the best of all possible type 2 worlds. If it *doesn't* work, or if it works for a while and then works no more, the next step is to use the pills we just discussed. These usually keep your blood sugar in the proper range for an average of five to seven years, although Virginia Valentine reports having one patient who's been successfully on the pills for twenty-five years.

Then, if the time comes that your physician decides that your blood sugars aren't what they should be—say, your fasting (before-breakfast) blood sugars are over 150 and your after-meal blood sugars are over 200—then it's time to call in the old master blood-sugar controller, insulin.

You may protest at this point, "I thought you said that I probably had lots of insulin floating around in my bloodstream—maybe even too much." You probably did have plenty of insulin. That's *did*. Past tense. Over the years your poor pancreas has been working overtime. Now it's weary. It can no longer produce enough insulin to keep your blood sugar in the acceptable range, so you have to help it out by bringing some more insulin on board.

Maybe your doctor will give you a combination of pills and a small amount of NPH—intermediate-acting—insulin at bedtime to see if that does the job. Other doctors believe that once the pills stop working you shouldn't use them anymore at all and will put you directly onto insulin alone.

Many type 2's who go onto insulin are put on only one shot of NPH a day. That's usually not a good idea because it probably won't keep you in control for the entire twenty-four hours. One of the better insulin-therapy programs currently being used is to take two shots a day of a combination of premixed 70 percent NPH and 30 percent Regular (fast-acting) insulin. This combination usually covers you all day and night and takes care of your after-meal blood-sugar rises as well.

We know you don't like reading about taking insulin. You don't even like to think about it. But really, taking insulin is not as bad as it sounds. Most people who've built it up into a horrifying monster are surprised that it's not such a big deal once they get into doing it. Actually, it even has an advantage beyond the obvious one of keeping your blood sugar normal and preventing complications. It costs a lot less than the pills.

Since being overweight is such a problem for type 2's, how can I lose weight quickly, easily, and permanently?

Before we get into that BIG subject, we want to explain why losing weight, no matter how you do it, will be a tremendous boon to you. Simply put, for type 2's it will decrease your insulin resistance and may allow you to give up pills or even insulin. Losing as little as 10 to 20 percent of your current pounds will give you much better blood-sugar control.

So how do you do it? You've no doubt noticed that there are as many schemes out there for losing weight as there are for getting rich quick. The secret is to find the method that works for you. (Oprah's way is not necessarily your way.) We'll lay out some of the options, but remember that many of the plans will promise you magical miracles, but most of them turn out to be blue smoke and mirrors—and expensive ones at that.

The Health Professional's Formula: The Low-fat Diet

You've all heard this one for the last decade. The dictum is that eating fat is what makes you fat. That's why the supermarket shelves are loaded with products labeled no-fat or low-fat and no cholesterol. This type of diet may have been prescribed for you when you were first diagnosed as an overweight type 2. Its guidelines are based on the U.S. government's Food Guide Pyramid, with fats, oils, and sweets at the top—with the admonition to "eat sparingly" of this group—and at its base the bread, rice, and pasta group, which is supposed to be the mainstay of your diet. It has been the diet preached to all overweight Americans, but by and large it hasn't worked well. For example, despite the popular acceptance of this diet, one-third of all Americans are now classified as overweight; that means 20 percent over their ideal weight. One reason it hasn't been very successful, in particular for type 2 diabetics, is because of their "thrifty genes" and overproduction of insulin within their own bodies. Health authorities often blame the dieters when this diet doesn't work, claiming that they've overeaten on everything but fat and consumed way too many calories.

The strict low-fat diet is now being modified, especially since research has shown that type 2's with high blood fats do better when they add more monounsaturated fats to their diet and lower carbohydrates.

The American Dietetic Association has even proposed a whole new strategy for weight control. The basic premise is that the dieter should forget the idea of "ideal weight" and stop trying to reach an arbitrary number on a standardized weight table. Focus instead on weight management. Their new program includes:

1. Your objective should be a healthy-for-you weight that can normalize blood sugar, blood pressure, and blood cholesterol.
2. It's better to lose a modest amount and maintain it for three to six months before trying to lose more. This may help your body adjust its metabolic rate.
3. How you feel and how much energy you have can be just as important a measure of success as a number on the bathroom scale.

Ann M. Fletcher, who interviewed two hundred successful dieters, reported in her book, *Thin for Life,* that most of her "masters of weight control" individualized the low-fat style: fruits and vegetables, small portions of lean meats or none at all, and lots of water but no fast foods.

Commercial Weight-Loss Programs

We must warn you that the restrictiveness of these systems almost precludes people from maintaining their weight loss. They just can't put up with the regimen forever. That's why the recidivism rate after five years is astounding.

Here are their basic plans:

Weight Watchers: low-fat and high fiber; weekly meetings; 50 percent carbohydrate, 20 percent protein, 30 percent fat; weekly fee $11–$13.

Jenny Craig: eat only their foods at first; weekly meetings; 60 percent carbohydrate, 20 percent protein, 20 percent fat; one-year plan $99; deluxe plan $349 a year.

Pritikin: five to six small meals a day plus aerobic exercise and strength training; 70 percent carbohydrate, 10–20 percent protein, 10 percent or less fat. This plan is similar to Dean Ornish's *Eat More, Weigh Less* diet, which is also 10 percent fat.

Diet Pills

The more precarious and sometimes medically dangerous way to go for a quick fix are such extremes as liquid diets and drugs. Fen/Phen has been recalled because of a potentially fatal heart-valve disorder it can cause. These can't be considered a lifetime solution and in most cases shouldn't even be considered a short-term one.

Exercise

We cannot praise exercise highly enough as the most potent solution to most weight problems. In combination with a good eating plan it is like a magic bullet. It is often the key to both weight loss and good blood-sugar control.

For a discussion of the pros of exercise, see pages 79–80; we might add here that recent research by kinesiology professor Katarina Bores of the University of Michigan has shown that women who walk for exercise become more sensitive to insulin if they walk at a relatively slow three versus four miles per hour. Best of all, at that pace they burn more body fat. A true case of less is more.

The Low-Carbohydrate Diet: A Diet of Last Resort

For a full discussion of this plan, see the special supplement at the end of the book.

Everyone talks about people with type 2 diabetes having to lose weight. I was diagnosed in my forties and told I have type 2, yet I've never been overweight in my life. In fact, I've usually been underweight. What am I supposed to do?

We know just how you feel. Your story is June's story. She was diagnosed at age forty-five and told she had type 2 diabetes, and she was thin at the time. After trying to make it on the pills for a year, she was actually gaunt because she'd been out of control for so long. When she went onto insulin—where she should have been in the first place—she regained her normal weight and health.

She and you are what is sometimes called type 1½, or what Virginia Valentine calls type 2-D, meaning deficient. That's because you're deficient in insulin. (She calls the other type 2's type 2-Rs because they're insulin-resistant.)

You have one foot in each diabetes world. You can be called type 2 because you were diagnosed in mid-to-late life, when most of them were. But then you could also be called type 1 because your pancreas doesn't produce enough insulin, so you'll have to take some insulin (better sooner rather than later like June). You won't, however, have to take as much as most true type 1's because you do produce some insulin of your own. Unlike type 2-Rs, your cells aren't resistant to insulin and you don't have a lot of insulin floating around in your bloodstream knocking on the cell doors trying to get in.

Incidentally, just last year June finally had a C-peptide test to find out just how much insulin she was producing. It turned out that she was producing no insulin; her pancreas had finally given up. Now she calls herself a true type 1.

For Family and Friends

They say that one person in four is touched by diabetes. That is to say, you have it, you eventually will have it, or you are a family member or close friend of someone who has it. Since you're reading this section, you probably fall into one of the two latter categories. And you have your problems, too.

June, in her more mellow moments, allows that she thinks diabetes is sometimes harder on family members and friends of diabetics than on the diabetics themselves. She may be right, especially when it comes to the parents of diabetic children. For many of them their guilt feelings, anguish, and constant worry are exquisite torture. Parents often lie awake fretting through the night while in the next room their diabetic child sleeps—appropriately enough—like a baby.

Some adult diabetics manage to lay all the responsibility for their care on a spouse. In these cases it's usually—but certainly not always—the wife of a diabetic who learns the diabetic diet, prepares it, and tries to see to it that her husband sticks to it while he remains aloof and unconcerned. On the other hand, we had a husband drop by a SugarFree Center who did the blood-sugar testing for his diabetic wife. He took the blood sample, read it, recorded the results—in short, handled everything—because she refused to have anything to do with it.

Friends of those with diabetes sometimes encounter the opposite situation. The diabetic person doesn't want to impose his or her problem on someone else and so will hardly talk about it, let alone clue in the friend on how to help on a day-to-day basis or even in time of emergency.

It's never easy. In a sense family members and friends are like insulin-taking diabetics who walk a tightrope between high and low blood sugar. Only the tightrope you walk is between not doing enough and doing too much, between being oblivious to a diabetic's problems and being concerned to the point of driving the diabetic—and yourself—crazy.

In this section we'll try to help you with your delicate and nerve-racking balancing act and show you that although you're touched by diabetes, you don't have to be pushed around, pummeled, and knocked out by it.

By the way, it's a good idea for you to read *all* the questions in this section, even the ones that on the surface don't appear to apply to you. You may find just the help you need buried in a seemingly unrelated situation.

Will diabetes make changes in our family life?

Only about as many changes as moving a hippopotamus into the living room. Each looms large on the scene, can't be ignored, has to be worked around, demands a great deal of time and trouble and care; and you never stop wishing that someone would take the damned thing away.

But strangely enough, you can get used to anything, be it hippopotamus or diabetes. Eventually when people express shock and concern—"Oh, you have a hippopotamus in your living room!" (or "Oh, your child, husband, or wife has diabetes!") "How terrible!"—you're surprised they even mention it as an oddity or a problem. It's just what *is,* a part of your life—and you're living with it.

How do I help the diabetic person in my life?

Learn. Learn all you can about diabetes. Become a walking encyclopedia of diabetes lore so you can be an intelligent and informed as well as a caring partner. Notice we say *partner*. Don't do it all. Don't try to take over. Don't make the diabetic—child or adult—totally dependent on you. That's not an act of kindness. People with diabetes have to be responsible for themselves. After all, you can't be around every minute—and even if you can you shouldn't be.

It's especially important for you to attend diabetes education classes and diabetes-association meetings with the diabetic person. Not only does this give emotional support, but two sets of eyes and ears absorbing the information make the program twice as effective.

If you have a diabetic child, we especially recommend that you join the Juvenile Diabetes Foundation International (see the directory of organizations in the reference section). Their primary goal is the worthy one of raising funds to finance research toward a cure for diabetes. But membership in this organization has the additional value of putting you in touch with other parents of diabetic children with whom you can share problems and—more important—solutions.

Another way to learn about diabetes is somewhat unusual, but if you're up to doing it, it will increase your understanding of diabetes tremendously and also help you develop empathy for the diabetic. Empathy is better than sympathy. Sympathy is feeling sorry for people; empathy is feeling how they feel, almost getting inside their skin.

Here's the way: You live exactly as a diabetic lives for a period of time. This idea was developed at the Diabetic Unit of the Queen Elizabeth II Medical Center in Western Australia, where they believed that the staff who treated diabetics needed to know what their patients' lives were really like. Volunteers for the experiment were required to take injections, using a saline solution instead of insulin, test their blood, eat the diabetic diet, including snacks at the proper time, etc. These educators had to "be diabetic" for only a week, but some of them couldn't last even that long. The only one who was really successful at it just gave up her social life entirely and stayed at home catering to her diabetes. That, of course, isn't the way to do it. You're supposed to lead a normal life. After all, that's the goal for diabetics, and that's what everyone else is always telling them they can do.

As Dr. Martyn Sulway, the physician in charge of the program, put it, "They found out having diabetes isn't a piece of cake." (Australian pronunciation: "pace of kaike.")

Barbara, even though she thought she knew all she needed to about the diabetic life, decided to try the experiment, because she'd been haranguing diabetics for years about what they ought to do yet had no firsthand experience. She did it, not for a week but for a month. It was a revelation.

Although she'd always bragged about eating the diabetes diet, she discovered that she hadn't been nearly as meticulous about it as a diabetic needs to be. For example, she hadn't always turned down *every* dessert. Also, she hadn't had to be continually worrying about keeping the inexorable snack on hand for an emergency, *and*—this irritated her the most—she hadn't had to eat when she wasn't hungry.

She took twice-daily blood sugars (and to her surprise discovered that she may have a twinge of reactive hypoglycemia). She took three injections a day. In order to have a little health hype out of it, she shot vitamin B_{12} instead of saline solution. Strangely enough, the injections weren't as bad as expected. At first they were an interesting novelty, but before long they became just a bore. Occasionally and for no apparent reason the shots hurt, but most of the time they were relatively painless.

She even managed to get the flu (not deliberately) and decided that if she really had been diabetic she would have wound up in the hospital because her diabetes-care program totally fell to pieces. This really brought home how important it is for a diabetic to avoid getting the minor diseases that go around every year.

Barbara also developed a greater tolerance for the foibles and peccadillos of diabetics. She has always been aghast at reports that some teenagers (and even one diabetic celebrity) shoot through their clothes when out in restaurants. But one night during the first week of the experiment she was dining out with friends and suddenly realized halfway through the meal that she'd forgotten to take her "insulin." So *zap!*— right through the old corduroy pants and into the leg. It turns out now that this is a common practice and it's okay to do it.

One of the worst features of "having diabetes," Barbara found, was having to keep your mind cluttered with it every minute. As June says, it's as if you're always playing an intricate chess game on top of whatever else you're doing.

The *truly* worst feature of diabetes—the worry about hypoglycemia and long-term complications—can't be duplicated in a nondiabetic person. Still, you can learn an amazing amount.

Why should I follow the diabetic diet and exercise plan?

It will help keep your diabetic loved one doing it. But that's not the main reason. The main reason is that it will maintain your own good health. There's nothing peculiar about the diabetic life-style. It's what we all should be doing. If you read the recommendations for good health from the Department of Agriculture and Department of Health and Human Services, or the American Heart Association, they're nothing more than the well-balanced meals with fresh fruits and vegetables, whole grains, and reduced fats that are recommended for diabetics. The diabetes exercise program, too—regular amounts of aerobic exercise and strength training—is exactly what everyone should be doing, according to all fitness experts.

Actually, having a diabetic person in your life or home is a tremendous boon. It wakes up the entire family to the best way of living and gives them an incentive for doing it.

It's particularly valuable when there are nondiabetic children in the family. If a sister or brother or parent has diabetes and the house is therefore bereft of junk food, they're going to develop healthy eating habits that will stay with them all through life.

Then, too, if any of the nondiabetics have the genetic gun loaded with a diabetic tendency, leading the diabetic life-style may well keep the trigger from ever being pulled.

And here's what may be the most effective inducement: If you have a diabetic spouse and he or she follows the diet and exercise program and you don't, you won't be able to measure up to your youthfully lean and vital counterpart. This can be bad for the dynamics of the marriage, to say nothing of your ego.

We feel compelled to warn you, however, of a built-in hazard when you're a nondiabetic in the company of a diabetic. That hazard is the old slip twixt the cup (and the fork and the spoon) and the lip. In other words, although you know better, you are constantly tempted to eat for two, and, alas, you often succumb to that temptation.

Here's how it works. The well-behaved diabetic is eye-measuring his or her food at a meal and eating right on the diet. You're doing pretty much the same, or maybe you're eating a *little* more, because after all you don't have to be all that careful with your measurements.

Then it turns out there are leftovers. They'll never be so tasty again. In fact, it would be foolish to try to keep them. And you don't want to waste all that good food. Think of the starving people around the world. So . . . down the hatch.

A few hours pass, and if the diabetic takes insulin it's time for a snack because he or she has to have small amounts of food at regular intervals to feed the insulin. As long as the diabetic is munching you figure you might as well be companionable and munch along. Your snack, which, again, doesn't have to be so carefully measured, goes down the hatch.

Dining out is even more tempting and hazardous. Perhaps there's a bottle of wine and the diabetic permits him- or herself one three-ounce glass. Somebody has to drink the rest. It cost a lot of money. You can't send it back, and they don't have doggie bags for liquids. Down the hatch.

Maybe there's a really fantastic dessert selection and the dessert comes with the meal. The diabetic prudently says no. Two desserts go down the hatch.

When you and the diabetic are at a friend's home for dinner, your eating for two becomes almost a social necessity. The hostess has worked so very hard on hors d'oeuvres and exotic concoctions—especially exotic dessert concoctions—that she's going to be wounded right down to the bottom of her saucepan if *someone* doesn't lap up with gusto everything in sight and ask for more. The diabetic can't. It's up to you. Down the hatch.

If this keeps up, before too long that hatch of yours is going to be attached to a tub, a tub that is in imminent danger of sinking. This is especially true if the diabetic person in your life is a relative, such as a sister or brother, with whom you share the same heredity. In this case, with your eating for two you could chomp your way into Diabetesland.

You have been warned. If you don't want that long and healthy life insurance policy your diabetic loved one has provided for you canceled, you have to pay the premium. That premium is to exert the same self-control as he or she and eat for only one. Then close down the hatch.

Should I marry someone with diabetes?

That, like the decision to marry at all, ultimately has to be your own decision, as you undoubtedly well know. The probable reason for asking this is that you're concerned about the problems your potential mate's diabetes might cause in the future.

It's wise to think about these possible problems now rather than later. As diabetes teaching nurse Diane Victor said to a young man who was complaining about some aspect of his wife's diabetes and shirking his responsibility for helping to deal with it, "Look, you knew she was diabetic when you married her. You signed on for the duration. Shape up."

Diabetes is never problem free, as we've made clear in this book and as you have probably already personally observed if you have a close relationship with a diabetic. Diabetes care takes time, time you would prefer to spend on more entertaining activities. Diabetes care takes money, money you would prefer to spend on other things. For a woman, diabetes can make having children more difficult, hazardous, and—again—expensive. And diabetes, if not cared for properly and controlled, can eventually cause debilitating complications and an earlier death.

But all of this doesn't mean you should give back (or take back) the engagement ring. Marriage is full of risks. You could marry a flawless specimen bearing a doctor's certificate of perfect health and the day after your wedding he or she or even you could get in an accident that paralyzed everything south of the earlobes. We have a friend whose apparently healthy wife developed multiple sclerosis in the first year they were married.

There are no guarantees in life. When you get married, the old "for better or for worse; in sickness and in health" still holds true. Realistically considered, diabetes, if well controlled, is one of the lesser worses and healthier sicknesses, and knowing about it in advance gives you a chance to learn and prepare and adjust.

Of course, it is possible for diabetes to destroy a marriage. Some marriages are so tenuous that they can't survive any adversity. In such cases, if it hadn't been diabetes that caused the breakup, something else would have.

Diabetes can also strengthen marriages. When one partner develops a potentially life-threatening condition, this makes the other realize how important the previously taken-for-granted person really is. Working together to control diabetes can, in fact, bring a new closeness. We heard of a long-married couple whose children had grown and who had gradually become so consumed by their individual interests that they hardly had anything left in common. Each was running on a separate track. When the wife was diagnosed diabetic, the tracks merged as they headed toward the same goal.

In the final analysis we believe that love conquers all. By this we don't mean the short-lived romantic love that turns your mind to irrational (but delicious) mush. No, we're referring to the enduring, day-to-day growing love that comes from living through and living with problems together and helping each other play out whatever hands you may be dealt, trying to turn the game into a winning one.

Does a diabetic child disrupt a family?

A diabetic child can disrupt it or can merely change it, in some ways for the better. Disruptions occur when the parents are filled with guilt, anger, or both. We heard of a husband who blamed his wife for the child's diabetes and threatened to divorce her "if anything happens to that kid." Obviously, he hadn't heard of the theory of the cause of type 1 diabetes being a virus, just as the cause of the measles or mumps is a virus.

Parents fraught with guilt can coddle and overindulge a diabetic child. This not only creates resentment and feelings of being unloved in any other children in the family but can be ruinous for the diabetic child as well. Diabetes can become for the child an excuse for dependence and manipulation of other family members instead of a stepping-stone to strength.

On the other hand, psychologist Barbara Goldberg, writing in *Diabetes Forecast,* emphasized that every family of a diabetic child that she talked to "mentioned that, in spite of, or perhaps because of, the illness, there was a special protectiveness, helpfulness, and a greater sense of family closeness."

This also holds true if one parent becomes diabetic. In American families these days we tend to be more than somewhat child centered. If a parent becomes diabetic and needs attention and care from the rest of the family, this develops in the children an increased responsibility and sensitivity to the needs of others.

In one family, the father, who had flexible business hours, spent much of his spare time chauffeuring the kids to their many and varied sporting activities and cheering them on from the sidelines. When he developed diabetes and had a need for exercise himself, the kids made it their business to see that dad got his jog every day and took turns accompanying him on it. New responsibilities. New closeness.

What can I do for my diabetic child?

There are many things you can do. You can help the child accept the disease and teach him or her how to take care of it. You can encourage diabetic children to achieve whatever they want to achieve in life despite diabetes. But there's one extremely important thing parents sometimes fail to do because they don't know it needs to be done—help diabetic children get rid of some of the terrible fears they carry around inside and suffer over and don't talk about.

Dr. Robert Rood, a San Fernando Valley diabetologist who works with children and adolescents, told a story about a child at a summer camp where he was serving as physician. This girl was a model camper, full of fun and very popular.

Dr. Rood, in checking out her blood tests, discovered that her one shot of insulin a day wasn't doing the job. (These were the bad old days when one shot a day was typical.) He decided to divide her insulin into two doses—morning and evening. This worked fine. Her blood sugar returned to normal. But *she* became very *ab*normal—sullen, negative, picking fights. When he took her aside to talk, she broke down and started crying. "I don't want to die," she said between sobs.

"Die?" said Dr. Rood. "Why are you talking about dying?"

"I know my diabetes was bad before when I had to take one shot. *Now* it must be getting lots worse because I have to take two. I'm going to die. I know it."

Dr. Rood reassured her, of course, and she became her old self again, but he had learned something important. You never know what's going on in a child's head. You have to take the time to talk and explain. Be especially careful if there are any major changes in diabetes routines, lest the child interpret them as Dr. Rood's camper did.

Diabetic children also sometimes believe their diabetes is a punishment for "being bad." This gives them guilt feelings as well as fear that if they're ever "bad" again something even worse will happen.

And don't overlook the hidden fears and guilts of the nondiabetic children in the family. Younger children can get the idea that when they reach the age when the older child got it, they'll get diabetes, too. Each day to them becomes like the tick of a time bomb.

Guilt feelings arise when nondiabetic children have harbored some quite normal sibling-rivalry evil thoughts, like "I wish Eddie would die," and lo, Eddie gets diabetes. They hold themselves responsible.

Parents must be aware of these dangers when the element of diabetes enters the family. Diabetes means there must be closer communication, more understanding, and more openness in the family. And that's all to the good.

What's it like to be a diabetic child?

First, let us give the view of a physician who deals solely with children. Dr. Lynda K. Fisher is at this time president of the ADA, Western Region, and director of the Department of Endocrinology and the Diabetes Division of Pediatrics at The City of Hope National Medical Center in Duarte, California. Dr. Fisher wrote the following article, "A Doctor Admires Families and Their Ability to Adapt," for the *Los Angeles Times* Health Section, November 24, 1997.

> I have spent the last twenty-two years caring for children and adolescents with diabetes, and I continue to be amazed, awed, and impressed by my patients and their families.
>
> Diabetes is a terrible disease, a chronic metabolic disorder for which there is no cure. The vast majority of people have the false perception that diabetes is not serious and that insulin injections (or,

for some people with type 2 diabetes, oral medication) are as good as a cure.

Not true. Inadequately controlled diabetes leads to blindness, kidney failure, heart disease, stroke, nerve damage, and limb amputations. However, the future of those with diabetes is not all bleak.

Results of a ten-year study reported in 1993 proved that if the blood sugars were kept near the normal range, the risk of developing the complications listed above were decreased by as much as 60 percent to 70 percent. Well, this sounds great, but it isn't easy and it is not fun. It is hard work, and the work never ends.

A day in the life of a child or adolescent with diabetes starts soon after waking, when he or she takes the first of four to eight (or more) blood tests of the day. Using a device that has a spring-loaded blade, he or she obtains a drop of blood, which is placed on a small, specially designed strip, which, when put into a glucose meter, indicates the level of glucose in the blood at that time.

The child with diabetes—or a parent or other responsible adult—then carefully measures the amount of insulin (the hormone that controls the flow of glucose into the body's cells) into a syringe and injects the insulin into the tissues under the skin.

One would think that this would be enough of a hardship for anyone, but it is just the beginning for a child, adolescent, or adult with insulin-dependent diabetes.

After taking the insulin injection, most children will wait fifteen to sixty minutes for the insulin to start working before they can eat breakfast. If their blood glucose was higher than the "normal" level, then they need to determine how much extra insulin they need and how much longer they need to wait to eat—while the rest of their family or friends just eat.

While at school, they need to worry about when during the day PE will be scheduled and how much activity they will have, as greater activity causes a more rapid and prolonged lowering of the level of blood glucose, which can lead to the annoying and often dangerous effects of hypoglycemia (low blood sugar).

Often, extra food needs to be eaten prior to increased activity to prevent low blood sugars even if the person is not hungry.

The child with diabetes and his or her parents must constantly survey their lives to search for events that may have an effect on diabetes—and there are many.

Once home from afternoon activities, youths need to decide whether the activity they just had will make them need to adjust their food for their usual insulin injection given at dinner time. Obviously, any activity after dinner can affect the amount of insulin required. If they want more food, they will need to take more insulin.

Now comes the often worst time of the day for parents of a child with diabetes: bedtime. How much insulin will be needed to control the diabetes and yet take into consideration activity level or potential changes in food? Does the child need extra food to prevent the frightening and often devastating complication of hypoglycemia, or extra insulin because the blood glucose level was too high?

Is the child at risk of developing low blood glucose and possibly seizures during the evening? Should he or she eat more, or take less insulin? Should he or she wake up in the middle of the night to check the blood sugar level?

And then: How does the child deal with parties and dances, and trips away from home? Who should he or she tell about the diabetes, and how much should they learn to help the child if needed?

So much to do and so much to learn! When you have diabetes, you become your own "doctor," in a sense, working with your doctor and diabetes team to control your diabetes.

What I have learned from my patients, and what is so awesome, is how well these children and their families do with all of these tasks. How well with the appropriate support they adapt these new requirements into their lives without giving up their lives. How much even young children know about their diabetes and how they teach and support others. How they do all of the things they need to do and get up and do it all the next day.

Diabetes is not fun, but new insulins, glucose meters, and insulin pumps now allow for easier care and increased freedom for people with diabetes.

The future is much brighter now that we know we can reduce complications, but it is not enough. It still takes too much work. We need a cure for diabetes, and that takes money for more research. Increased dollars were set aside this year by Congress and President Clinton, but it is not enough. We all need to do more. (Reprinted with permission.)

And here is the story from the point of view of a thirteen-year-old girl, Erin Harris, who lives in southern California, and wrote, to go with Dr. Fisher's article, the following article of her own, "A Teen Becomes Her Own Physician, Always on Call."

When my dad asked if I wanted to write an article about what it is like to have diabetes, I hesitated.

I am not ashamed of having diabetes, but it brings no great joy to my life either. It does make me different, and I like to be discriminating about whom I can trust about something so personal.

I finally decided to do this because so many people are so clueless about the disease. One of my mom's friends is certain that I will outgrow it, and another recommends that I use herbal insulin therapy to avoid toxicity . . . whatever that means.

I find most general health care professionals have little training in the field and are not astute about the everyday workings of diabetes.

So, what is it like to live with diabetes?

Maybe the better question is: What is it like *not* to have diabetes? My condition was diagnosed when I was four. I have a faint memory of intense thirst and getting up all night to urinate. I remember my mother sobbing into the night. I thought I did something horrible to make her cry like that. I recall thinking, "Why is everyone around me so sad?" I could not understand what was happening. It's not easy giving your pinkie to poke when you are four years old.

Guess what? It's no different at thirteen.

I do not remember not testing my blood sugar every morning, noon, and night. I do not remember not taking insulin injections, sometimes three times a day. I do not remember going to the refrigerator and taking any little thing my little heart desired without a voice that said, *"Warning."*

Not to say that I'm not tempted sometimes. The consequences are more than I care to think about. My endocrinologist is always reprimanding me to record my blood sugars so that my insulin doses can be adjusted. It really sucks!

Inasmuch as my life differs from my friends' lives, technology allows me to do more than ever before. I enjoy all sorts of rigorous activities, from karate to dance. I play the piano and love to read.

And along with insulin therapy comes retail therapy. You guessed it. I love to shop. I consider the mall a major physical workout. I simply have to take a little more time and calculate my activities into my food and insulin regimen.

Consistency is essential in maintaining normal blood sugars. I am certain my parents will confirm that I am consistent at doing the mall.

I am beginning to realize that I have to swap spontaneity for good health. It gets to me sometimes, especially when eating out or at a party and I am surrounded by M&Ms that are calling my name.

Generally, I feel grateful to be living in a time when there is a treatment for what ails me. Though there is no cure, I pray for the courage and strength to take me through whatever lies ahead. I live with the continuous hope that the cures for diabetes as well as all other illnesses are just around the corner.

My parents, family, and friends are very supportive. My father, Dr. Michael Harris, is a board member of the American Diabetes Association. Together, we spend much time and energy trying to raise money and make others aware that there are sixteen million people walking around with diabetes—and half do not know they have it or what it could do to them.

That, ladies and gentlemen, is scarier than my sister's room. (Reprinted with permission.)

If my diabetic child goes to a birthday party or trick-or-treating on Halloween, is it all right to break the diet just this once?

Think how many "just this once's" that would make in a year. Before long, just this once becomes an everyday occurrence, and bad habits are established. Your child's health and maybe even life expectancy are diminished.

It's hard to see your child deprived when other kids are loading up on goodies—maybe it's even harder on you than on the child—but diabetes is going to be there all his or her life. Now is when lifetime behavior patterns are established. You're *not* being kind when you let your child break his or her diet just this once.

One thing you can do on occasions when your child is being deprived is figure out some way he or she can get extra attention. Attention is an even more satisfying commodity to the young (or the middle-aged and old, for that matter) than ice cream, cake, and candy. Let your child pass out the forbidden food to others in much the same way that some alcoholics like to act as bartender at parties.

You can also give parties at your own home. That allows you to present approved food in such entertaining ways that neither your child nor the guests will realize, or care, that they aren't getting the junk food their hearts desire.

As for Halloween, your first decision is whether to allow your child out at all. If you do, and he or she comes home with a bag of loot, ADA board member Netti Richter, writing in *Diabetes Forecast,* offers some good suggestions:

> Why not help sort out the acceptable healthy foods and save a few sugary ones for handling reactions? What about the rest of the candy? In our house the garbage disposal is a great eater of "nondesirable foods."
>
> Knowing that resisting candy will be rewarded by an exchange gift at evening's end might make trick-or-treating less frustrating for a child. For example, exchanging the candy for a Halloween storybook at bedtime can be fun.

Use your own imagination to help your child stay on the diet instead of using your pity to allow him or her to break it "just this once."

Now, after having given the official party line, which happens to be our own opinion as well, here's a more lenient variation reported by a physician whom we respect, Dr. Lawrence Power, author of the syndicated column "Food and Fitness" and consulting physician for National Health Systems (publishers of health reference charts).

A colleague of his who sees many diabetic children and young people says that a number of young diabetics, especially teenagers, who don't want to be different and who long for the fun foods their peers get to wolf down, totally rebel. They refuse to follow their diets and as a result stay constantly out of control.

This doctor makes a deal with the kids. If they promise to stick to their diet at all other times, they get six Hog Wild Days a year, six celebration days such as Christmas or their birthdays or graduation day, when, as far as food is concerned, anything goes.

"Do you know how high they usually kick up their heels on those days?" the doctor asks. "A Coke and a hamburger or a hot fudge sundae. Big deal."

Dr. Power himself adopted the Hog Wild Day method with his adult heart-attack patients. "Everyone needs a binge now and then," he says, "whether it's mint bonbons, Big Macs, or a cholesterol quiche. Something in most of us calls for a break from the routine. . . . There's room for the occasional departure for a holiday. It is the daily habits that get us into health mischief, not the occasional celebration."

Only you know your child well enough to decide whether the Hog Wild system would be a safety valve that would let off enough steam to allow him or her to simmer down to a good daily dietary routine or if it would only break down the already flimsy barriers against hazardous eating habits.

If you *do* opt for Hog Wildness, you should have a clear understanding with your child that the six days are to be spread out over the year and not clustered into an orgy week that could prove disastrous.

Should I send my child to diabetes summer camp?

Unless your child is the kind who would be miserably homesick and suffer psychological damage at *any* summer camp, we think it's a good idea—especially for younger and newly diagnosed children. We've had reports from young people who consider their camp experience a breakthrough in understanding their diabetes and in learning new practical techniques of management. Even more important to them was the realization that they're not oddballs and that the world is full of other diabetic children who are successfully coping with the condition.

It's a genuine comfort for a diabetic person to be in a situation in which virtually everyone has diabetes and the person *without* diabetes is the peculiar one. Barbara experienced this one day back when we ran the SugarFree Centers. June and Ron, both diabetic, were on the scene, as was our cleaning woman, also diabetic. (We practiced reverse discrimination and hired diabetic employees whenever we could.) Everyone who came in had diabetes. All the mail was from people with diabetes. Barbara began to get the creepy feeling that she was the only nondiabetic person on earth and that there was something wrong with her for *not* having it.

Summer camp is also a good way for a child who has perhaps been overprotected at home because of diabetes to develop self-reliance.

One major benefit of diabetes summer camp is for the parents. For a short while you get out from under the stress and strain of worrying about your diabetic child. You know he or she is in the best of hands and you can get away for a little R and R yourself. You need it and you deserve it. Stress works its damage on you as well as on the diabetic child.

Summer camp can also give you a chance to improve your relationship with any nondiabetic children in the family. They may be developing feelings of being less loved because they don't get the constant concern that the diabetic child gets. A week or two of exclusive attention can be a booster shot of security and self-esteem for them.

We have heard a few complaints about diabetes summer camps, including one from a mother whose already too-thin child came home five pounds lighter and showing ketones, and from a young woman who was disturbed and disgusted by the wild goings-on with alcohol and marijuana in one camp for teenagers. But these are isolated instances. The overwhelming majority of the reports have been favorable. There is one summer camp for the entire family, where five or six families with diabetic children are brought together in eastern Maine for a week. It is described in Dr. Joan MacCracken's book, *The Sun, the Rain, and the Insulin* (see the reference section).

What can we do if we can't afford all the costs involved with our child's diabetes?

There is help available in the form of Supplemental Security Income (SSI). This is a federal program that makes monthly cash payments to disabled people who don't own much in the way of property or other assets and who don't have much income. Diabetes counts as a disability. A child's SSI payment can be as much as $477 a month, although some may get less because of their parents' income.

For further information, and for instructions on how to file, call the SSI office at 1-800-772-1213.

I just can't get my husband to take care of his diabetes no matter how hard I try. Is there anything I can do?

Unfortunately, you're not alone. Many people are desperate about trying to get those they love to take care of their diabetes and themselves. We frequently receive letters like the following, written by a young man:

> I have been involved with a wonderful lady name Sheila. About a year and a half ago we learned that she is a type 1 diabetic. We are always considering marriage, but I must admit I'm frightened about our future together. Her problem is not the fact that she is diabetic. She has been fighting a losing battle with a severe sugar addiction. It has nearly destroyed our relationship many times, and she becomes so depressed that it is really unbearable. She desperately wants to beat this addiction to sweets, but nothing has seemed to work for more than a day or two at a time. There is some progress, but I fear that time is quickly running out. Sheila has already noticed a decrease in her vision as well as constant poor circulation. Her diabetologist dropped her as a patient because she was not doing what he told her. It's evident that these sugar binges of hers could prove fatal.
>
> I love Sheila with all my heart and soul and want so much to beat this damned disease and have as much of a future as God would permit us. Such a wonderful person as Sheila deserves as full a life as possible. I hope she can take control of this disease before it takes control of her.

We also get success stories. We received this note attached to a law school graduation announcement: "We got our meter in December. Since then my husband's diabetes has been controlled. It certainly took a load of worry off my mind during my last year in law school. In that light I wanted to share my graduation with you."

One young woman confessed to us that her husband told her that she used to be disagreeable about half the time, but since she started controlling her blood sugar, she's become "a wonderful human being and a joy to be around."

You might have your husband read the preceding so he could see what a shattering—or positive—effect a diabetic's control can have on loved ones. You could express your feelings. Even if he isn't willing to control the diabetes for himself, he might start doing it to free you and the rest of the family from worry and allow you all to live your lives to the fullest.

But if people with diabetes should decide to control their blood sugar for the benefit of others, they should also investigate why they don't want to control it for themselves. Don't they consider themselves worth the effort? Don't they love themselves enough? If the answer is no, they may have a real problem, a problem more serious than diabetes and one for which they should seek professional counseling.

But if your husband still won't take care of himself, remember that it is as Dr. Richard R. Rubin says: "Nobody can make anyone else do something they don't want to do." He advises you to "recognize, grieve, and finally accept the reality of your own limits." But still, "you should never stop trying new ways of helping the person locate his or her own motivation for change."

What is this "honeymoon period" I hear about?

This can occur in type 1 diabetes—particularly in children—shortly after insulin treatment begins. The diabetes seems to be in remission. Less insulin, or sometimes none at all, is needed for diabetes control. This often causes parents who are already desperately clutching at straws to think their child has been miraculously cured or that the diagnosis was wrong. False hope. Diabetes is still there. A remission is not a cure and should never be regarded as such. Enjoy it while it lasts, but realize that it will end, and don't let yourself be devastated when it does.

My wife wants to think and talk about diabetes all the time. What can I do?

It's hard to find a person with diabetes who's middle-of-the-road. Either they try to ignore the disease totally or become almost obsessed by it. Those who fall into the obsessive category are at least better than the ignorers. They'll probably live longer and eventually outgrow their obsession.

As a matter of fact, many people are obsessed only for a while, right after they're diagnosed. It's not surprising that they should be preoccupied when they first confront a disease that demands the constant attention and thought that diabetes does. Much of the diabetic's talk about diabetes at this time is just musing out loud as he or she tries to figure out what to do.

One way that might tone the diabetic decibels down a little is to become more informed about diabetes yourself. By showing that you know something about the subject, your wife may begin to feel less desperate about the subject and relax and let you do some of the thinking. If the two of you have workable give-and-take exchanges on new solutions to diabetic problems, perhaps she will be able to cut the personal, lonely fretting time in half and start to think and talk about something else.

Your advantage in knowing about diabetes is that when it's the subject under discussion, you'll understand what's being said. Then the talking will seem a lot less like a foreign language you don't speak, and, consequently, it will become a lot less boring to you.

If this plan doesn't work or just seems to feed the obsession, you may eventually have to express a little tough love. Say in no uncertain terms that nobody loves a monomaniac and that such obsessive behavior is only going to alienate people. This won't be easy for you to do, especially since you're so full of sympathy and love. But unless somebody delivers the truth, your wife is going to have a blighted life, always feeling—and behaving—more like a walking case of diabetes than a human being with infinite interests and infinite possibilities who just happens to have diabetes.

How can I tell if a diabetic person has low blood sugar?

It helps if you know the person well enough to recognize behavior that isn't normal. If a generally easygoing person starts snapping and snarling, it may be low blood sugar. If a decisive person becomes vague, that can be a clue. Fumbling hands, glassy eyes, slurred speech, perspiration on the forehead or upper lip, a dopey smile, an odd, taut look about the face—all can be symptoms of hypoglycemia. Just about all diabetics have some signs peculiar to themselves that you'll grow to recognize if you're around them a lot and are observant.

Even if you know the person well, though, it's not always easy to recognize low blood sugar. We still remember the time we were talking to the Glendale chapter of the Diabetes Association of Southern California and told about one of our editors who said she could always recognize when June had low blood sugar "because she starts being mean to Barbara." We noticed a woman in the audience frowning. During the question-and-answer period she said, "My little boy has diabetes and takes insulin. Often, in fact, *very* often before dinner he's a holy terror. I can't do a thing with him. Could that be low blood sugar?"

"Oh boy, could it!" we chorused.

She was really shaken, because she had been punishing him for what was probably a misbehavior of his chemicals.

When you ascertain that a diabetic person does have low blood sugar, take action immediately (see pages 142–143). Above all, don't follow the example of the sister of a diabetic friend of ours, who, when she saw he was starting to act funny, looked terrified and announced, "You've got low blood sugar! I'm getting out of here!" And she fled.

How can I keep from getting mad at my roommate when he's obnoxious because his blood sugar is low?

It's tough not to get mad. You're human, too, and sometimes you have a visceral reaction that you can't control. Just do your best to keep calm enough to help your roommate get out of the reaction, even if he fights you on it.

After the incident is over you'll probably both laugh about it. Once June had low blood sugar and became furious because she thought Barbara had eaten her dish of strawberries (which she had actually eaten herself, but couldn't remember). After her anger came despair, as she wept over her disappointment about the strawberries she had so looked forward to. With a baleful look at Barbara, she kept wailing, "You stole my strawberries." Throughout all this wrath and woe, she steadfastly refused to eat anything else to bring up her blood sugar because "the only thing I wanted was those strawberries and you ate them." In retrospect, the incident seems funny to us, but while it was going on it was like a scene out of Eugene O'Neill. At such times you feel you're dealing with an insane person. (Of course, you are.) So never take seriously or bear a grudge over something a diabetic person says or does when in hypoglycemia.

You have one big advantage in this situation: You know what low blood sugar is and can usually recognize it. This puts you way ahead of the average person. Think how people who know nothing about diabetes must react when confronted by your roommate's obnoxious behavior.

*I don't like to be impatient with all the things my wife
has to do to take care of her diabetes, but I admit that
sometimes I am. Is there anything I can do about it?*

All of us with diabetic friends or family members want them to take
good care of themselves and stay healthy so we'll enjoy their love and
companionship for years. And we know that taking care of diabetes
takes time—lots of it. We know this intellectually but not always emotionally. For example, sometimes we're ready to go out to dinner or a
movie or a sports event, and we have to stop and wait for a blood-
sugar test or a snack or some diabetic something-or-other. We may get
impatient, even irritated. We're not upset with the diabetic *person,* of
course. It's the diabetic *condition* that bugs us. Still, the diabetic person
is receiving a negative message, even if it's being delivered in a silent
language.

You don't like yourself for your impatience with diabetes routines,
but you can't help it. Or can you? It's possible for you to turn these moments of time that diabetes steals from you into moments that you steal
for yourself. All you have to do is figure out some things you really want
to do, and reserve these stolen moments to do them. You can read a
book. You can work a crossword puzzle. You can play a musical instrument. You can do needlework. You can meditate. You can practice magic
tricks. You can do anything that doesn't take a lot of time to set up.

If you get in the habit of truly enjoying the diabetic-routine time,
it will help both you and your wife be happy. You may even start hearing yourself say to her, "Are you sure you don't want to test your blood
sugar before we go out?"

*What am I likely to do that will irritate my diabetic
husband most?*

Remember the old Paul Simon song, "Fifty Ways to Leave Your Lover"?
Well, there must be 150 ways to irritate your diabetic husband. In fact,

if your husband is an insulin-taker and gets low blood sugar, anything you do, including trying to get him to eat something to raise his blood sugar, is likely to bring on anything from irritation to a full-blown rage. (Some diabetic people in the throes of low blood sugar have even been known to hurl food into the face of the person trying to help.)

All persons with diabetes, even when their blood sugar is normal and even if they don't take insulin, have their pet peeves. You'll just have to find out with experience what they are.

We can start you off with a few tips, though. A diabetic person hates to hear the same phrase over and over from you. For example: "Is that on your diet?" "Did you remember to take your injection?" "Did you bring along a snack?" Anything you keep repeating begins to grate after a while.

June, for some reason, gets furious when asked, "Do you have low blood sugar?" (She claims Barbara always asks this in an accusatory tone.) Her response is usually a garbled conglomeration of "How should I know?" "Do you see a blood-sugar sensor sticking into me that I can read?" "Do you want me to stop what I'm doing and take my blood sugar; is *that* what you're saying?" Rant. Rant. Rant. She actually prefers to be told, "You're acting weird" or asked, "Why are you being so obnoxious?" probably because it's not the oft-repeated phrase that she's come to loathe.

Nagging, which one psychologist defines as "trying to control with criticism," is also near the top of the diabetic irritation scale. Nagging is not only irritating but also futile. As we've repeatedly pointed out, changes are only going to be made when the diabetic person wants to make them. The best you can do is help him truly accept diabetes and to find the motivation to make the necessary changes. (See pages 35–36, "How do I start making all the changes I have to for my diabetes?")

Another thing that will bother your diabetic husband is your cadging snacks. Insulin takers need to carry sweets and other foods at all times in case of a reaction. If those who are aware of this rich storehouse of goodies persist, like Goldilocks, in eating them all up, the diabetic person can be in deep trouble in an emergency when, like Old Mother Hubbard's, the snack cupboard is bare.

A far, far better thing to do is find out what your husband likes for low-blood-sugar snacks and carry those yourself for diabetic emergencies—and for your own snacking pleasure.

But probably the number one irritant for diabetic people is a lack of effort on the part of intimates to understand diabetes. Among June's close friends are some she's known for years and in whose homes she's frequently had meals. They have supposedly read most of our books, and yet they still have only a vague idea of what she can and cannot eat. They understand little about how her meals must be scheduled or what to give her when she has low blood sugar. Since these friends are not stupid, she can only infer that they don't really care. A feeling that your friends don't care goes deeper than irritation. It goes into the hurtful-wound area.

As an appropriate finale to this discussion, here are Dr. Richard Rubin's "Ten Commandments for Avoiding Negative Scenes with Diabetic Loved Ones," reprinted from his book, *Psyching Out Diabetes:*

1. THOU SHALT NOT ACT LIKE A POLICEPERSON. This approach doesn't work and can ruin your relationship.
2. THOU SHALT NOT IGNORE DIABETES. Don't expect your loved one to carry on all activities as if the diabetes did not exist.
3. THOU SHALT NOT LEAD YOUR LOVED ONE IN THE PATHS OF TEMPTATION. Many diabetics find it upsetting to be constantly face-to-face with forbidden fruits, and they often get angry at the person who's eating those fruits in front of them.
4. THOU SHALT NOT CRITICIZE WHEN YOUR LOVED ONE SUCCUMBS TO TEMPTATION. Sure, you're frustrated, but adding insult to injury is a surefire argument starter.
5. THOU SHALT NOT TALK ABOUT YOUR LOVED ONE'S DIABETES IN PUBLIC UNLESS INVITED TO DO SO. Public comments tend to be taken as criticism, so take your cue from your loved one.

6. THOU SHALT OFFER SUPPORT AND COMFORT, ESPE-CIALLY WHEN THINGS AREN'T GOING WELL WITH THE DIABETES. For any number of reasons, diabetics are often very touchy when their control is bad. A little extra TLC goes a long way toward avoiding confrontations at these times.

7. THOU SHALT HAVE THE PATIENCE OF A SAINT WHEN YOUR LOVED ONE IS ACUTELY HYPO- OR HYPER-GLYCEMIC. These can be the worst of times, and if you both lose your heads . . . More on this issue later.

8. THOU SHALT DEAL CONSTRUCTIVELY WITH YOUR OWN NATURAL FEARS AND RESENTMENTS. Your diabetic loved one is not the only one living with the disease. You are, too, and you will feel scared, angry, even overwhelmed at times. You must find a way to deal with these feelings constructively, on your own and with your loved one. The key is to acknowledge what you're feeling and to take responsibility for the feeling. Some of the suggestions for doing this, made earlier in this chapter, might help.

9. THOU SHALT BE ESPECIALLY SENSITIVE IN PUBLIC SITUA-TIONS. Eating right, testing, and taking shots can be especially stressful for diabetics in public settings, so your diabetic loved one might be edgier than usual. Be alert for opportunities to make things a little easier.

10. THOU SHALT FIND OUT WHAT WORKS AND DO IT. In your family, a number of diabetes-related situations may often lead to conflict; for instance, when your loved one has high blood sugar, eats something he or she shouldn't, or fights you when you want to help him or her deal with an insulin reaction. Find out what your loved one wants you to do in these situations, and do it. Don't wait until you're in the middle of a battle to ask, though. Ask when you're both feeling comfortable and relaxed. I never cease to be amazed at how well this simple approach works to avoid fights.

If I mention my friend's diabetes in a restaurant to try to get her something special, like a substitute for sweet-and-sour pork in a Chinese dish, she gets furious and says I make her feel like a freak. What can I do?

The answer is simplicity itself. You say to the waiter, "I am a diabetic and I can't eat anything with sugar in it. Could we please substitute pork with Chinese greens for the sweet-and-sour pork?" By claiming to be the diabetic yourself, you take the burden of asking for special favors off your friend's conscience, or pride, or whatever area of her psychological being is disturbed.

After you've claimed to be the diabetic for a while, maybe your friend will awaken to the fact that having diabetes is nothing to be ashamed of. She will come to realize that for the most part, people in restaurants as well as in other walks of life are usually happy to help out with little problems associated with diabetes. This is an important step in her acceptance of the disease.

What should I do if we're out dining in a restaurant and my brother, who is diabetic, orders all the wrong things?

People with diabetes sometimes perversely do this. Even June, who is the most careful and rational of beings, has occasionally suffered this restaurant aberration.

The best thing to do when you hear the diabetically inappropriate meal being ordered is *not* to screech and rant and embarrass your brother in front of the waiter, but rather to order a diabetic backup meal for yourself. Very likely, when the meal is presented to him, he will take one look at it and come to his senses. Then you just say casually, without any lectures or recriminations, "It looks as if my dinner might be better for you than yours. Would you like to trade?" He probably will, with gratitude, as much gratitude for the freedom from lectures and recriminations as for the food itself.

Naturally, to perform this little sleight-of-plate act, you have to know what a diabetically appropriate meal is. So read the diet section of this book, beginning on page 40.

How do I plan a meal for my diabetic mother-in-law?

Just remember that she has to stay away from concentrated sweets—sugar, honey, and molasses in or on foods, and canned fruit in sweet syrup. Many people also have to restrict the amount of fat they eat. Ask her. Remember also that those who take insulin need a specific amount of carbohydrate in their diet. Just have something like bread, rice, pasta, or potatoes available, and she will know how much of it to eat.

That's another point to remember. Just as important as what is allowed is how much. People with diabetes must eat limited quantities of food. Don't be offended if your mother-in-law eats with gusto and then suddenly stops, as if someone has blown a whistle. There isn't a bug in the food or anything. It's just that she has eaten all that's allowed. Don't urge her to have more. She would probably love to eat more, and it's taking every ounce of willpower to resist your elegant cuisine.

A basic diabetic meal would be something like this: a mixed green salad; chicken or fish or meat; potatoes or bread or pasta or rice; a vegetable or two; and fruit for dessert (either fresh or canned without sugar). Depending on which diet she's on, she'll have plenty to choose from.

Should I give up eating pastries so my diabetic sister won't feel tempted?

Admittedly, it's a little hard to sit there and wolf down a huge slab of banana cream pie if your sister is watching you like a spaniel. You both feel sorry for her, you feel guilty, and these are very digestion-upsetting emotions. Still, you definitely shouldn't give up your pastries for your sister's sake. She is going to have to get used to being tempted and resisting temptation. It's similar to the situation faced by alcoholics: They have to be able to go to a place where others are drinking and yet not drink themselves.

There remains, however, a question you didn't ask. And that is, Should you give up pastries for your own sake? Pastries are hardly the nutritional dream dish for anybody, diabetic or not. Your sister may guide you to good health and good looks.

My son wants to play football. Is that safe for a diabetic person?

There have been several outstanding diabetic football players. Ron Mix of the University of Southern California and Coley O'Brien of Notre Dame are just two. Many high-school football players shared their experiences with us when we were writing our previous books. No diabetic evil ever befell them because of football. If your son's diabetes is without complications and under good control and his doctor doesn't disapprove, then there is no reason he shouldn't play.

There are two good reasons he should. Participation in sports, especially a physically demanding one like football, will encourage him to take superb care of himself and his disease. For a young person, the incentive to keep in shape for football is far more powerful than a general incentive to watch one's health. Once your son has established good habits during his football-playing days, there's a fair chance he'll stick with them throughout his life.

He should be allowed to play football for psychological reasons as well. If his diabetes keeps him from playing football, he'll get the idea that because of diabetes he can't do anything.

On the other hand, if he plays football, his attitude will more likely be that, despite his diabetes, he can do everything he really wants to. Which attitude would you prefer him to carry through life?

Be sure he informs the coach and his teammates that he has diabetes and explains to them what they should do in case he has an insulin reaction.

And finally, do your best not to show excessive concern every time he goes out to play, even if you feel it way down inside your own pancreas. If you load him up with fears and negative feelings, you'll wreck his game and maybe cause an accident rather than prevent one. A football player needs a positive attitude above all else, and so does a diabetic.

Note: One case in which we feel you're justified in forbidding your son to play football is if your family doesn't believe in the violence of the sport and none of your children is allowed to play it. In that case it would be wrong to bend over backward and let your diabetic son do something you don't let the others do.

This same advice holds for a daughter who wants to participate in somewhat hazardous sports like ice hockey or downhill ski racing. In fact, she may need extra support because in her choice of sport she will be bucking both convention and diabetes.

Should I give my brother his insulin injections?

Yes and no. Yes, you should give them to him sometimes. You can reach injection sites he can't reach himself, unless he's a contortionist. This is a big help.

Another reason for giving him his insulin is that you'll know how to give an injection. Should he ever pass out in insulin shock, you'll know how to give him glucagon (see pages 144–145), which is injected in the same way as insulin, and bring him out of it.

But no, you shouldn't *always* give him his injection. He's got to be mainly responsible for his own insulin shooting. No one should be that dependent on another person. It's almost like being dependent on another person for your breathing. It's not good for him or for you, either.

What's the best way to celebrate my diabetic partner's birthday or other special occasion?

It takes some ingenuity and foresight to create the kind of birthday celebration that's best for a person with diabetes. Fortunately, there are now sugar-free baking and frosting mixes available. If you keep those on hand, you'll always be ready to make something for birthday parties and other special occasions. Check with the local bakeries. As part of the diabeticization of America that we've been talking about, many bakeries are adding sugar-free cakes to their repertoires. (We know of four in the Los Angeles area.) You can even be truly original and make something like a sandwich cake. It looks like a cake, but when you cut into it, it's actually a club sandwich frosted with something like blended cottage cheese and yogurt.

When it comes to gifts for diabetics, you should heed the excellent advice given in the journal *Diabetes Self-Management,* by Charles Mallory, a Kansas City free-lance writer who has a diabetic wife:

> Don't make every gift related to diabetes. Treats don't always have to be sugar-free candy or dietetic chocolates, nor does a Christmas gift have to be a health-club membership or dinner out at the new low-calorie restaurant. Your wife probably likes flowers, traveling, clothes, and entertaining. Your husband may like cufflinks, cologne, or a greeting card for a special occasion. None of these has to do with diabetes. Wouldn't you be disappointed if, at a birthday party, your friends who knew you were Catholic gave you nothing but Virgin Mary statuettes and rosary beads?

What should I do if I were to find a diabetic person unconscious?

Unconsciousness can be due to either diabetic coma, which means the person has extremely high blood sugar, or insulin shock, which means it's extremely low. If you know that person takes insulin and sticks to his or her diet pretty well, then you can be almost certain it's insulin shock.

First, never under any circumstances pour any liquid like fruit juice or Coca-Cola down an unconscious person's throat, as it could wind up in his or her lungs and cause suffocation. The only thing you can do, if you've had good instruction and know where it is, is give an injection of glucagon. Otherwise, call the paramedics or a doctor. A word to the thrifty: an injection of glucagon costs about $40; calling the paramedics can cost over $400.

If you know for sure that the person doesn't take insulin and/or doesn't follow the diet or take care of him- or herself, then it's probably a diabetic coma, the result of poor diabetes control over a long period. In this case, call the doctor or an ambulance immediately. There's nothing much you can do in this kind of crisis. Only a hospital can help now.

If you have no idea whether you're dealing with insulin shock or diabetic coma, treat for insulin shock. If it's diabetic coma, the person already has so much sugar floating throughout his or her system that a little more isn't going to make all that much difference. And if it *is* insulin shock, your quick treatment could be a lifesaver. A person in good health will eventually come out of insulin shock spontaneously, but for someone with a heart condition the shock could be life threatening.

The Diabetic Dietary Court
of Last Resort: The
Low-Carbohydrate Diet

"God help us when doctors disagree."

—ANTON CHEKHOV, *UNCLE VANYA*

There is nothing on today's diabetes scene that generates more disagreement and confusion than diet. Many people ask us, "How do you know what's the best diet to follow when there are conflicting opinions from experts?" In our answer to this we cite Chekhov's statement. It also holds true for disagreeing nurses, dietitians, psychologists, exercise therapists, and others.

What to do? Since God helps those who help themselves, we each have to find out what works best for us. As one correspondent, Beth A. King, said, "Strange how diabetes is like fingerprints. No one has the same symptoms or results."

Fortunately, we have the tools to find out what works best for us: scales to see if our weight goes up or down, testing equipment to see how our blood sugar is affected, laboratory blood tests to see what happens to our cholesterol and triglycerides. Plus we can see how we feel on the diet. Are we energetic? Sluggish? Ebullient? Despondent? In the end we have to be the ones responsible. Diabetes is like that.

THE ANTHROPOLOGICAL
SIDE OF DIET

How were we human animals meant to eat? What diet will keep us healthy? The anthropologists disagree as much as Chekhov's doctors. Try these opposing quotes:

From *Reversing Diabetes* by Julian Whitaker, M.D.:

> Most of our degenerative diseases in this country can be traced to our meat-based diet, and diabetes is no different. An animal protein diet is just plain wrong for the human system, which is designed for the clean-burning carbohydrates and fiber found only in vegetable foods.

From *Protein Power* by Michael Eades, M.D., and Mary Dan Eades, M.D.:

> Most experts agree that game-hunting was the primary means of sustenance for our ancestors. Natural selection molded our physiology to function optimally on a predominantly meat diet supplemented with roots, shoots, berries, seeds, and nuts.
>
> The change to the agricultural diet created many health problems for early man. The fossil remains tell us that in preagricultural times human health was excellent. People were tall, lean, had well-developed, strong, dense bones, sound teeth with minimal, if any, decay, and little evidence of severe disease. After the advent of agriculture and a change in diet (from 75 percent of calories from meat to only 25 percent) this picture of robust health began to deteriorate. Postagricultural man was shorter, had more brittle bones, extensive tooth decay, and a high incidence of malnutrition and chronic disease.

Hmmm. Well, moving right along, let's look into the history of the low-carb diet as far as people with diabetes are concerned.

SOMETHING OLD IS NEW AGAIN

Dietitian and diabetes educator Betty Brackenridge in her *New Nutritional Guidelines* audio tape (see the reference section) points out that back when insulin was discovered in the early 1920s,

> diet became precise prescription, an exact number of calories usually coming from a very low carbohydrate one, with little or no bread, potatoes, etc. And absolutely no sugar. It was thought that since the problem was an excess of sugar in the system, withholding sugar and other carbohydrate would make that problem easier to control. The difficulty was that there are a limited number of sources for food energy or calories. If you eat less carbohydrate, you're going to have to eat something else and that something else turned out to be fat.
>
> After some fifty years of being in vogue, low carbohydrate diets began to lose favor, when the relationship between a high fat diet and heart disease became known. So over the next twenty-year period we had various versions of a high carbohydrate diet with emphasis on high fiber sources of starch, a continued restriction of sugar, and some fine tuning of the types of fat in the diet to control various blood fats that are associated with heart disease risks.

A shadow of disrespectability was also cast on the low-carbohydrate diet by a number of low-carbohydrate diet books with titles such as *The Drinking Man's Diet* and *Martinis and Whipped Cream*. These titles alone made it sound as if no seriously health-conscious person would even consider a low-carbohydrate diet.

In the early 1980s, Herman Tarnower's less frivolous-sounding *The Complete Scarsdale Medical Diet* climbed onto the bestseller list. We were surprised to discover in the biography of Julia Child, *Appetite for Life,* that about this time she became interested in the low-carb, high-protein diet. Previously she'd never had any problem with weight. She could eat anything she liked, and her over-six-foot frame had always stayed svelte. She once gained eight pounds after a pasta-eating trip to Italy, but those were quickly gone when she got back to her normal eating pattern. But when she had a mastectomy and gave up smoking, she put on ten pounds. After taking these ten pounds off, she put on twenty. Later on, when she decided once more to lose weight and went on a twelve-hundred-calorie diet, she again lost ten pounds and put on twenty. (Sound familiar?) Inspired by her hairdresser's success on the Tarnower diet, she turned to the low-carbohydrate, high-protein diet and restored herself to her former slenderness. She continued to keep the weight off by following her "everything, but in moderation" policy.

The Scarsdale Diet died out after Tarnower was shot. (The perpetrator was not a disgruntled dietitian as one might suspect from the ire that this kind of diet incites in health professionals.)

Now the low-carbohydrate diet is starting to emerge into the sunshine of respectability again with books by Robert Atkins, M.D., Michael and Mary Dan Eades, M.D., and, specifically in the field of diabetes, Richard K. Bernstein, M.D., and Calvin Ezrin, M.D. (See the reference section for descriptions of these books.)

A DIETARY ODYSSEY

When June was diagnosed diabetic over thirty years ago, she followed the standard middle-ground diabetic diet and was in pretty good control. Then along came the Pritikin program and Dr. Anderson's HCF (high-carbohydrate, high-fiber, low-fat) diabetic diet, which had great appeal for her. This was, after all, the late sixties, when everyone was eating this way and grains and beans and vegetables abounded in restaurants with natural wood interiors, waitresses wearing saris, and a whiff of incense in the air. This diet seemed the healthy way to go. After all, it was only logical that the low fat would keep your veins and arteries unclogged and thereby keep cardiovascular problems at bay. For diabetics, the low fat had an additional purported benefit of making your insulin work better.

Nondiabetic Barbara, who, like every normal American woman, wanted to lose five to ten pounds, looked forward to seeing them melt away as she downed mounds of brown rice and beans of many colors. The low-on-the-food-chain, almost (or totally) vegetarian diet even made you feel virtuous. You were making the world a better place as you made yourself a better person.

At this stage in our odyssey we often merrily harangued—in letters and in person—our friend, Dr. Richard K. Bernstein, about the low-carbohydrate, high-protein diet for which he was a voice crying in the diabetic wilderness. (His rationale was that since it's the carbohydrates in food that are converted directly into glucose, beware of them.) We called his diet "unhealthy and immoral" and accused him of thinking only of normal blood sugars while ignoring the rest of a person's well-being. We even condemned him—although not to his face—of thinking that "all the world is Bernstein," and we said to each other that just because his weird diet worked for him didn't mean it would work for anyone else. Unfazed by our jocular criticism, he kept firing back scientific articles that substantiated his theories. Dr. Bernstein also suffered the opprobrium of his medical colleagues, one of whom told us, when we cited Bernstein in one of our books, "Bernstein is a very unreliable source."

The HCF diet worked for June for a while, but then her blood sugars started heading north, so she reluctantly slacked off the ultra-high-carbohydrate diet, still keeping the low-fat aspect. (Since Barbara had never lost an ounce on the diet, she, too, started backing off it.) June followed this more middle-ground dietary pattern with moderate success until her insulins of choice—beef Ultralente and purified pork Regular—were taken off the market after the introduction of human insulins because not enough people used animal insulins to make it financially feasible for the companies to produce them. On human insulins her blood sugars got increasingly out of whack.

About this time we were working on a new edition of *The Diabetic Woman* with Lois Jovanovic-Peterson, M.D. June's assignment was to transcribe one of the doctor's audio tapes on diabetic pregnancy. In these tapes the doctor described how she put pregnant women on a high-protein, low-carbohydrate diet so their blood sugars would stay normal for the benefit of the baby. June, disgusted with her diminished control and wanting to take care of her own "inner child," decided to see if a high-protein, low-carbohydrate diet would fix up her errant blood sugars. She was further influenced by the growing acceptance in the health professional community of "carbohydrate counting" as a way of stabilizing blood sugars. (If carbohydrate counting comes, can the low-carbohydrate diet be far behind?)

Simultaneously—and independently—Barbara, whose weight had "ballooned" to 116 pounds after a pasta and pizza orgy trip to Italy, decided she had to Do Something, and the low-carbohydrate, high-protein diet was it.

To our amazement and delight, the diet did exactly what we wanted it to do. June's blood sugars got almost boringly normal. Barbara immediately lost six pounds and within a few months lost five more, making her only two pounds over her lean college weight.

What about our blood fats? Haven't they gone stratospheric? Dr. Bernstein maintains that if your cholesterol and triglycerides are normal, they'll stay about the same. If they're high, they'll probably go down. That held true for us. June was already better than normal and stayed that way. (HDLs over 100, triglycerides under 40. Barbara's HDLs improved from 54 to 85; her triglycerides remained in the low forties. *(But you should keep having tests to make certain bad things aren't happening to your blood fats on the diet.)*

Even when we saw the results of the blood tests, we still had the question "Why?" We're eating more fat than before—especially more animal fat, including cheese and egg yolks. After all the screechings about fat causing high cholesterol that we'd heard—and believed!—we couldn't understand why the traditional view was wrong. It didn't make sense.

It's wrong, the low-carb books explain, because the more carbohydrate you eat, the more insulin your body must produce to cover it. The more insulin in your bloodstream, the more cholesterol is produced. To control cholesterol, you must therefore restrict the amount of carbohydrate you eat, and that in turn will reduce your insulin output. This truth is particularly valid for type 2 diabetics who have both overproduction of insulin (hyperinsulinism) and insulin resistance. For type 1's, the low-carbohydrate diet allows them to shoot up less insulin and have more normal blood sugars with the same cholesterol-lowering results. (And as a dividend, there are fewer of the incidences of low blood sugar that heavy doses of insulin can promote.) Here's another conundrum for you:

HOW CAN I LOSE WEIGHT BY EATING FAT?

Yes, yes, we've heard it over and over again like a mantra, Fat makes you fat. Fat makes you fat. Fat makes you fat. The new books explain that one, too. Eating fat is not what makes you fat. On the contrary, it's eating too much carbohydrate that does it. Carbohydrates are what make you fat because they cause the body to release more insulin, and insulin is a potent fat-building hormone. This is the premise, also, of Barry Sears's Zone diet.

Health professionals are still for the most part adamantly opposed to the low-carb diet. In fact some grow quite emotional about it. One dietitian even asked to have her name removed from our *Diabetic Reader* mailing list, saying, "Your publication does terrible things to my blood pressure, and my doctor has forbidden me to read it ever again." Why do they get so upset? One physician who is a proponent of the low-carb diet says it's because "it negates everything they have learned—and taught!—over their careers. It's profoundly threatening to them."

Some of the more broadminded dietitians say, in effect, "Okay, try this crazy diet if you must, but under no circumstances stay on it over six weeks." Dr. Bernstein has been following it for twenty-six years and just received a Joslin award "for courageously living with diabetes for fifty years."

THINKING ABOUT THE LOW-CARBOHYDRATE DIET: THE CONS OF IT, THE PROS OF IT, THE READY-SET-GOES OF IT

The low-carb diet is definitely not for everyone. There are several categories of people for whom it is not the highway to health and happiness. Check and see if you fit into any of these con categories.

THE CONS

You Don't Need It

If you have excellent control and are living joyfully and healthily on the mainstream diabetes diet, or the high-carbohydrate, high-fiber, low-fat diet, don't mess with success. Keep on keeping on. These two diets are generally recommended by health professionals, so you can experience warm feelings of approval and support when you report to their office. On these diets no one will shriek at you the way they will with the low-carbohydrate diet, saying that you're insane, you're clogging your arteries with cholesterol and making yourself a heart-attack candidate, and you'll probably develop osteoporosis and may even open the door to cancer. Why unnecessarily subject yourself to that?

You Shouldn't Try It

If you have kidney damage or gout, this diet isn't appropriate or approved because of its greater protein content.

You Can't Fit It into Your Life and Life-style

The low-carb diet may not be all that easy to fit into your life and the lives of your family. Those who don't have the goad of diabetes control or weight loss may not be willing to make the sacrifice of giving up cherished foods like pizza and pasta and popcorn and milk and cereal and fruit and juices.

This diet can also take more time to plan ahead and prepare than higher carbohydrate diets. In her pre-low-carb days Barbara wouldn't even think about lunch until it was time to eat. Then she'd rummage around the kitchen and dredge up some high-carbohydrate food like popcorn and milk or a peanut butter and something-or-other sandwich. Now she has to be certain to have protein and lots of it on hand. It's often a challenge.

This diet is expensive. When we asked one of the doctor proponents of it which people should not go onto the diet, he ticked off those with severe kidney damage, those with gout, and (pregnant pause) paupers. Of the three dietary elements carbohydrate, fat, and protein, protein leads all the rest in cost. That's why in Third World countries people eat very little protein. It's used more like a seasoning, and carbohydrate—lots of it—is the dietary staple.

You Have Ethnic Dietary Reluctance

It would be very difficult if not impossible for a card-carrying Italian to give up pasta, polenta, risotto, and the delicious Italian breads. Most people of Asian descent couldn't imagine a meal that didn't include rice. And how would people of Mexican heritage feel about a meal without tortillas or beans? The list goes on and on from country to country around the world. If, because of your upbringing, when you have a meal without your obligatory ethnic carbohydrate you feel you haven't eaten at all, then no matter how much good this diet might do for you, it ain't gonna happen.

You Can't Even Stand the Thought of It

If this diet is totally repugnant to you, it would be a waste of time to even think about following it. Let's put it this way. What if you were absolutely, positively guaranteed that you could live to be 150 and every moment of that life you'd be completely free of any and all diseases and disabilities of mind and body, and then you would die quietly, peacefully in your sleep surrounded by loving family and friends? Sounds good, doesn't it? But there's a catch. To make this happen you'd have to follow an unusual diet. Would you do it? "That depends," you would logically say. "What's the diet?" Every day for the rest of your life you would have to eat a cocker spaniel. We don't know anyone who would do that no matter what the benefits would be. The low-carbohydrate diet is to many people as unthinkable as a cocker spaniel a day. They're going to have to find other routes to control and weight loss.

The diet could repel you for a couple of additional reasons:

You're a Vegetarian

You may be a vegetarian because you don't believe in eating animals, because, in a world of hunger, you feel it's immoral to eat so high on the food chain, or both. But a vegetarian for whatever reason would have a great deal of difficulty following this diet. As Dr. Atkins says, "It's theoretically possible to construct a healthy low-carbohydrate vegetarian diet, but there aren't a lot of foods on it. The narrow range of foods is too boring." If you can't have your protein in beans and grains—as you can't on this diet—and you can't drink milk because of the carbohydrate, you may grow weary of eggs (or egg substitutes) and cheese and tofu. Even if you're a real tofu hound, it might not work out well for you because, as dietitian Dr. Linda Sherman points out, tofu protein doesn't stay with you as long as animal protein.

Her recommendation for patients who are vegetarians is to change their mental set and to think of animal protein not as food but as medicine. Another of the tricks of her trade is to see if there is any animal protein they're willing to try for just a week. Sometimes they will say they might be able to handle some fish or chicken. She says those who do try it generally feel so much better and see such good results that they stick with the diet despite their initial reluctance. Linda, incidentally, has a great deal of empathy for vegetarians because she was once one and would still like to be one. As she says, "my heart and mind are vegetarian, but my body is low carbohydrate, high protein."

We've checked around to find a really-o, truly-o vegetarian who is following and enjoying the low-carbohydrate diet. So far we've found no one. But if you're a vegetarian and go onto the diet, please let us know so we can pass on the how-to-do-it information to others.

You're a Fatophobe

There are a lot of Jack Spratts among us who can't stand fat—especially animal fat—in any form. It makes them literally and figuratively nauseated. This may be something physical or something psychological or the way they were brought up, or it may be because it's been drummed in their dear little ears by health professionals and health writers and friends and relatives and even casual acquaintances that fat is the next worst thing to poison and is bound to result in obesity and an early grave from horrifying maladies.

It *is* possible to avoid fat on this diet. Dr. Calvin Ezrin, author of *The Type II Diabetes Diet Book,* in particular, explains how. A certain amount of fat goes with the high-protein territory, but this is not an impossible situation. If you're clever and conscientious, you can pretty much have it both ways: low carbohydrate/high protein/*relatively* low fat, avoiding animal fat when possible. June's a semi-fatophobe and she's managing it.

THE PROS: WHY YOU MIGHT CONSIDER THE LOW-CARBOHYDRATE DIET

Unlike the many cons—why you shouldn't or couldn't go onto the diet—the pros are a very short list of two.

It's the Dietary Court of Last Resort

You've honestly and sincerely made a great effort to control your blood sugar and/or lose weight on the middle-ground diabetic diet or the high-carbohydrate, low-fat diet. You've done it over a period of time. More likely you've done it over and over and over again over many different periods of time. And you've failed over and over and over again. You've probably been accused of "cheating" because nobody could believe that if you religiously followed one of the more conventional diets and you did your exercise as prescribed, you wouldn't lose weight. Virtually all the experts and their books say you will. But you didn't (cheat) and you don't (lose weight). What's wrong with you?! Nothing. (Except, of course, diabetes.) And the low-carbohydrate diet may prove that to you.

It's a Diet You Could Love

For years you've been a good boy or girl trying to do the best for your health. You drink nonfat milk although you think it tastes like chalk. You chose margarine over butter although you detest margarine and worry about the chemicals in it. You always order low-cholesterol egg substitutes. You've almost forgotten what a slice of real bacon looks like. Now, suddenly, you're presented with a diet that turns the food pyramid upside down and turns old enemies into friends and vice versa. One diabetic man—actually a doctor—was virtually vegetarian for years. When he couldn't keep his blood sugar under control, he experimented with the low-carbohydrate diet, and it worked for him. "But," we asked him, "how are you handling all the protein and fat if you're a vegetarian?" "I was only a vegetarian because I thought I should be for my health. I'm having a ball with this diet!" A French friend, Marguerite, had failed to lose weight and lower her blood pressure on the high-carbohydrate, low-fat diet prescribed by her HMO. Her daughter, an avid low-carber, convinced her to switch. Not only was it effective for her, but the cheeses and patés and roast meats she loved had been returned to her. As she says, "Now I'm laughing all the way to the refrigerator."

Barbara—a true daughter of the Midwest—who grew up savoring barbecued ribs and bacon and cream and fried-just-about-everything is now in—well, let's face it—hog heaven.

If you're a closet protein and fat lover, this "medicine" can turn out to be nectar for you, and you can finally eat, without embarrassment or apology, what you've really wanted to all along.

THE READY-SET-GOES

Helping Hands

If you've decided to give the low-carbohydrate diet a try, you shouldn't try to do it alone. You need the aid and comfort and guidance of your health care professionals. This is true for all diabetics but particularly so for type 1's, whose blood sugars may plummet rapidly on the low-carbohydrate diet and who will need help in insulin adjustment.

Most health professionals, even if they don't personally believe in the diet, are willing to help you try it for a short while, "maybe a month," to see if it works. They're usually even more willing to participate in the experiment if they've seen you struggle with your blood sugar or your weight and seen you fail. They know—and share!—your discouragement and frustration. If there's even a chance this could be the answer to the unanswerable, then why not see if it is?

Helping Pens

Along with the helping hands of your health care team, you need to have some helping pens—books and tapes by people who've been there and done that low-carbohydrate diet. And you'll need reference books to help you learn the carbohydrate values. *You can't follow this diet with books alone, but it's very hard to follow it without books.* You need them on hand for when you're confused and to give you confidence and facts and figures in the face of the barrage of verbal slings and arrows you'll get from people who think this diet is nutty and dangerous.

Helping Internet

If you want to prowl the Internet for low-carb lore, the first place to go is LC-DIABETES, Grant Magnuson's "support list for all persons controlling intake of carbohydrates as a method to manage diabetes and avoid diabetic complications. . . . The purpose of the list is to share experiences, offer each other support, chat about our daily challenges in the spirit of sharing knowledge on dietary and health issues of our chosen life-style." Grant does, however, sound a cautionary note: "Information obtained from this list might not be accurate or medically appropriate for everyone. Each reader must draw their own conclusions about how to use any information obtained from this list. Each reader must do their own analysis of any claims made. In all cases it is recommended that people consult medical professionals on a regular and timely basis." To join up, send e-mail to LISTSERV@maelstrom.stjohns.edu with the message: SUB LC-DIABETES Your Name. Or visit: http://www.mountain-inter.net/~magnuson/.

Another Web page on the low-carb diet that is not specifically related to diabetes is The Low Carbohydrate Diets Information Center: http://people.delphi.com/elizjack/.

Helping Newsletter

Twice a year we publish *The Diabetic Reader,* and in that we always include an update of information on the low-carb diet recipes and sources for such low-carb foods as crisp breads, tortillas, and protein bars. To receive a complimentary copy, call 1-800-735-7726 or e-mail prana2@aol.com or write to us at 5623 Matilija Ave., Van Nuys, CA 91401.

EASY DOES IT!

One of the reasons we like this diet is that it's so easy to follow. You really only have to think of one thing: carbohydrates. No more fiddling around with all those exchanges, which are inaccurate anyway. (For example, all bagels are not created equal, and neither are all apples.) And there's no more figuring and juggling the proteins and calories and fat and carbohydrates in the food you eat, as June tried to do in her beginning days of diabetes.

At first you do have to do measuring and weighing and calculating, but soon you'll have the basic carbohydrate values in your head and will be able to eyeball portion sizes fairly accurately.

The diet depends on counting carbohydrates so you can eat the exact number of grams you need to for each meal. Yes, you must get into gram counting, even though we Americans do not use the metric system and are not very familiar with it. Like the British, we generally measure in ounces. An ounce is equivalent to approximately thirty grams; to complicate things just a tad, food portions are usually measured in ounces. For example, eight ounces of milk (one cup) has twelve grams of carbohydrate. Therefore, you need to know both your portion size and its number of grams of carbohydrate for all foods you're planning to eat. Fortunately, the many food analysis guides, plus the labels on supermarket products, do most of the job for you. (See the reference section.)

Most low-carbohydrate diet books also have good lists of foods and their carbohydrate content. Sometimes these are classified according to the number of grams of carbohydrates. For example, they'll have lists of five-gram portions, lists of ten-gram portions, etc. Another method is to tell you the percent of carbohydrate in each food. In that case, you weigh your portion in grams, multiply it by the percent of carbohydrate in that particular food, and, voilà, you know the amount of carbohydrate in that portion. For instance, strawberries are only 0.08% carbohydrate. Let's say you weigh four large strawberries and they're 120 grams; multiply this by 0.08 and you get 9.6 grams of carbohydrate.

Since May 1994, new federally mandated nutrition labels appear on all packaged food products. (The government does *some* things right!) These labels tell you both the number of grams and the percentage of carbohydrate per serving.

To summarize, you need a good carbohydrate guide, a hand-held calculator, and a food scale that gives both grams and ounces. It won't take long for you to build up your personal memory bank of the carbohydrate content of foods—especially your favorite foods—so you can eat with confidence at home and in restaurants.

OUR WAY

We're telling you how we handle the diet *not* to suggest that you do it the same way, but to show you how simple and easy the diet can be. You'll want to do what we did: read books and choose what's best for you. Your diet will probably be, like ours, an amalgam. What we do is a less meticulous Bernstein (for example, we have occasional small servings of low-carb fruits such as canteloupe and strawberries), Ezrin with more fat, Atkins with caffeine, and Eades without dietary vacations. Unlike all of them (except Bernstein), after over three years we still haven't upped our carbohydrates in a maintenance program. Many followers of the low-carb diet, after achieving their goal of weight loss and/or blood-sugar control, gradually increase the carbohydrate in their diet until the goal starts slipping away. Then they drop back into the safe zone of carbohydrate consumption for them and there they stay.

Thirty Is the Magic Number

We eat a total of thirty grams of carbohydrate a day. June, as Bernstein recommends, divides it into six at breakfast and twelve each at lunch and dinner. She never saves up carbs from one meal to the next. Barbara sticks to thirty but, as a nondiabetic, is more casual about their distribution and does put some in her carbohydrate bank to use later in the day—but not from one day to the next.

We exercise thirty minutes a day, usually beginning with stretching and hand weights (for upper-body strength) and following up with either a walk, a workout on the exercycle (June), or a treadmill trot (Barbara).

We each drink thirty glasses of water a day. Just kidding. But we do try to drink as much as we can hold. That's an important part of the diet, especially in the early stages. Since it's hard to get down as much water as you should, we try to remember to drink a glass of it about half an hour before each meal. (Insulin takers could drink it when they take their pre-meal insulin.) This not only gives you automatically three needed glasses of water but also fills you up so you don't need to eat as much at the meal. This is particularly beneficial for those trying to lose weight.

As for the protein, we follow the Bernstein suggestion of eating an amount that allows you to leave the table feeling comfortable but not stuffed. We also go with his idea of keeping the size of the protein portion at a particular meal constant from one day to the next. This means that "if you eat six ounces at lunch one day, you should have six ounces at lunch the next." (He considers this especially important if you're taking blood-sugar-lowering medications.)

We pretty much let the fat fall where it may. You can let your conscience and your blood chemistry tests be your guide on the type of fat—and how much of it—to incorporate into your own diet.

And that's it. But don't necessarily do as we do. Do as we say. With the help of your diabetes health care team find your own unique low-carbohydrate path to blood-sugar control and/or weight loss and—surprise dividend!—increased energy with no midmorning or late-afternoon slumps. Dr. Bernstein says that the diet also improves your memory—although we haven't noticed so far that it has.

SOME PRACTICAL MATTERS

Going Shopping: A Positive Approach

We were planning to visit a friend for a few days. He was totally flummoxed about what to cook for us on our "strange diet," especially when we started rattling off the things we couldn't have. But happily in *Dr. Atkins New Diet Revolution* we found a terrific list of what we *could* have. With this positive approach, our friend relaxed. "Why, you can have *everything!* It will be no problem at all to cook for you."

We initially planned to send you to the market to browse and read the nutritional information on the packages and come to the chilling realization that it's a carbohydrate jungle out there. Now we know better. Go positive shopping. Fill your cart with a plenitude of noncarbohydrate and low-carbohydrate foods. You'll be astonished at the choices. Don't think restrictions; think opportunities to try a new variety of delicious foods.

PROTEIN AND FAT FOODS
(called "Free Foods" by Dr. Atkins)

MEAT	FISH	FOWL
Beef	Tuna	Chicken
Pork	Salmon	Turkey
Lamb	Sole	Duck
Bacon	Trout	Goose
Veal	Flounder	Cornish Hen
Ham	Sardines	Quail
Venison	Herring	Pheasant
in fact, all meat	*in fact, all fish*	*in fact, all fowl*

SHELLFISH	EGGS	CHEESE
Oysters	Scrambled	Aged and Fresh
Mussels	Fried	Cow and Goat
Clams	Poached	Cream Cheese
Squid	Soft Boiled	Cottage Cheese
Shrimp	Hard Boiled	Swiss
Lobster	Deviled	Cheddar
Crabmeat	Omelets	Mozzarella
in fact,	*in fact,*	*in fact, almost*
all shellfish	*all eggs*	*all cheeses*

Exceptions: 1) luncheon meats with nitrites or sugar added
2) products that are not exclusively meat, fish, or fowl, such as imitation fish
3) all cheeses have some carbohydrate and quantities are governed by that

SALAD VEGETABLES
(10% CARBOHYDRATE OR LESS)

Alfalfa Sprouts	Endive	Parsley
Arugula	Escarole	Peppers
Bok Choy	Fennel	Posse Pied
Boston Lettuce	Jicama	Radicchio
Celery	Mache	Radishes
Chicory	Morels	Romaine
Chives	Mushrooms	Sorrel
Cucumber	Olives	

VEGETABLES IN ADDITION TO
SALAD VEGETABLES

Artichoke Hearts	Christophene	Sauerkraut
Asparagus	Collard Greens	Scallions
Avocado	Dandelion Greens	Snow Pea Pods
Bamboo Shoots	Eggplant	Spaghetti Squash
Bean Sprouts	Hearts of Palm	Spinach
Beet Greens	Kale	String or Wax
Broccoli	Kohlrabi	Beans
Brussels Sprouts	Leeks	Summer Squash
Cabbage	Okra	Tomato
Cauliflower	Onion	Turnips
Celery Root	Pumpkin	Water Chestnuts
Chard	Rhubarb	Zucchini

The Fabulous Fiber Freebie Trick

After you have a handle on the foods you can have on this diet, then you should prowl the supermarket aisles to see if you can expand your choices by finding products with a high-fiber content. In her lucid and authoritative audio tape *Carbohydrate Counting* (see the reference section) dietitian Betty Brackenridge explains how fiber lowers the total carbohydrate count of foods:

> Fiber is technically a carbohydrate, but people can't digest it, so it doesn't produce any blood sugar. It's as if it weren't there for the purposes of carb counting. For most foods the amount is small—one or two grams and you can just ignore it—but for high-fiber foods, those that contain five or more grams of fiber per serving, you should subtract the grams of dietary fiber from the total carbohydrate.
>
> For instance, the label on a high-fiber cereal like Fiber One says it has twenty-four grams of total carbohydrate in a one-half-cup serving, but it also has fourteen grams of dietary fiber in that same serving. If you counted the whole twenty-four grams, you'd be overestimating the cereal's effect on your blood sugar by over one-half. When you subtract the fourteen grams of fiber from the twenty-four grams of total carbohydrate, you get a much more modest ten grams of carbohydrate for each one-half cup of Fiber One, the amount that's actually going to impact on your blood sugar. If you use the total carbohydrate content without subtracting the fiber, you might overestimate the needed insulin dose or underestimate your carbohydrate intake by enough to cause low blood sugar in the middle of the morning.

What this means to low-carb dieters is that fiber is one of your best friends, as it is both "free" and healthful. All people are, in fact, advised by dietary experts to eat a minimum of twenty to thirty-five grams daily. If you seek out extra fiber, it will not only make it possible to add more carbohydrate to your diet with impunity, it will take care of the complaint of the anti-low-carb-diet contingent that the diet doesn't contain enough fiber. It also takes care of another complaint we've occasionally heard from some followers of the diet: constipation. With more fiber, more water, and that thirty minutes of exercise a day, constipation should never be a problem.

Note: For the low-carb diet with its strict counting of grams, you should subtract even small amounts of fiber from the total carbohydrate content of a food.

When you browse the market aisles armed with your knowledge of this trick of deducting the fiber from the carbohydrate, you can expand your diet more than you thought possible. Alexandra, an enthusiastic low-carbing friend, does this and as a result discovered Dr. Vogel's Mixed Grain bread (available only in Southern California, alas) and Indian papadums, a kind of cracker that puffs up all crispy in the microwave, and even some dark chocolate–covered almonds from See's Candy (another Southern California favorite) that weigh in at only three grams of carb per piece. Every week she finds some more affordable—in the low-carbohydrate sense—treats, and so can you in your part of the country. Let us know what you find, and we'll spread the word.

Some of the Best Things in Life Are Free

Well, these aren't exactly the *best* things in life, but it's a comfort to know that when you really feel you want something and you've used up all your carbohydrate allotment you can still have: coffee, tea, diet sodas, sugar-free gelatin (in Dr. Bernstein's early days of the low-carb diet, he used to eat a quart of it a day!), celery, and the old George Bush favorite, fried pork rinds, also known by the more exotic and appetizing name, *chicharones,* which you can use for dipping. These last give you that much-longed-for crispy crunch that you used to get from things like potato chips and popcorn in your pre-low-carb days of yore.

The Low-Carb Breakfast of Champions

There is an old saying, "So much depends on breakfast," meaning that the outcome of the day is influenced by a good start. But followers of the low-carb diet could reverse that to "Breakfast depends on so much": so much planning, so much shopping, so much preparation, and—most important—so much adjusting your thinking as to what breakfast should be.

We receive a multitude of questions about what you can have for breakfast on this diet, hearing such plaintive wails as, "If I see another egg, I'm going to start cackling." Fran McCullough in her *Low Carb Cookbook* (see the reference section) recognizes the breakfast problem, saying, "In some ways, this is the most difficult meal of the day." But if you really get into making minor adjustments and attitude changes, it can turn out to be the most exciting and tantalizing meal of the day.

One of the things people start missing right away is sitting down to a quick bowl of cereal. The good news is that it needn't be lost. Just crumble up two or three Bran-a-crisps, sprinkle them with a low-carb sweetener like DiabetiSweet, perhaps add some cinnamon and a few chopped nuts, and pour cream over it all. If your carb allotment permits a bit of a lower-carb fruit, strawberries or raspberries are a delicious addition.

At first contemplation of the low-carb diet's restrictions, you would logically think that your classic and cherished Sunday morning pancake breakfast will be forever denied you. Not so. We've evolved a recipe for . . .

Low-Carbohydrate Sour Cream Pancakes

½ c. sifted soy flour   ⅔ cup sour cream
¼ tsp. salt   2 slightly beaten eggs
¼ tsp. baking soda

Sift flour, salt, and soda together. Whisk together sour cream and egg. Pour into the sifted flour mixture and gently stir only enough to moisten the flour. No beating!

Heat a nonstick griddle or skillet (with a little vegetable oil, such as peanut or avocado oil, if you don't mind the extra fat). Drop the batter onto the pan by generous tablespoons. When you see bubbles on the tops of the pancakes, turn and cook on the other side. Serve with sugar-free, low-calorie syrup. A tasty variation is to add chopped nuts to the batter.

Makes eight 3½″ pancakes (two servings). Each serving = 288 calories, 10 grams carbohydrate, 13 grams protein, 18 grams fat.

Before going onto the low-carbohydrate diet, June used to love to bake. The process was good for her mental health, and the results made for mealtime delight. Scones were her favorite breakfast treat. She was heartbroken when she felt her scone-baking days were over. But with luck and pluck and imagination and soy flour she was able mend her heart by creating low-carb scones just as good as the ones of yesteryear—maybe even a little better.

Pecan Cream Scones

1 c. soy flour	½ c. lightly toasted chopped pecans
1½ tsp. baking powder	½ c. cream
½ tsp. salt	1–2 tbsp. melted sweet butter
5 packs DiabetiSweet	1 tsp. lemon zest

Preheat oven to 375°. Sift together flour, baking powder, salt and DiabetiSweet. Add the chopped pecans to the dry ingredients. Add the lemon zest to the cream and pour into the dry ingredients. Mix lightly until just barely combined.

Divide the dough into two balls. On a lightly floured surface, knead slightly. Roll one ball into a one-half-inch-thick circle. Cut like a pie into five pieces. Place each piece on a Pam-sprayed baking sheet about one-half inch apart. Repeat for the second ball. Paint the top with melted butter and bake 12–15 minutes until golden. Remove from baking sheet immediately and cool on a rack.

Makes ten scones. One scone = 141 calories, 4 grams carbohydrate, 3.6 grams protein, and 10 grams fat.

To get more adventuresome, you can try some international favorites (only the British seem to be as addicted to the bacon-and-egg breakfast as we are). On a bike trip through Holland, we quickly became fans and followers of their breakfast table of cold cuts: cheese, ham, and various other meat products along with the occasional optional boiled egg. This fortified us for the strenuous day ahead, and if it was a truly heavy day on the road we could even eat a bit of the gingerbread we purloined from the breakfast table.

In Norway they fueled the ski tours with a selection of cheeses, smoked fish, and marinated herring. Yes! Herring for breakfast. In sour cream it's particularly good.

In Germany, specifically in Munich, they have what they call *Zweites Frühstück* (second breakfast) in midmorning—usually *Weisswurst* (a white veal sausage) and beer. You could easily have this for your *erstes Frühstück* (first breakfast), grilling any kind of sausages you can find in your local markets—especially the ethnic ones. Since beer is pretty high carb (except for Miller Lite, with 3.2 grams) and it is pretty early in the morning, better skip the beer component of the meal.

The Japanese breakfast is composed of a variety of fish and seaweeds and small salted plums, all served up artfully and beautifully on plates of different designs and colors. When we were in Japan, Barbara always ordered the Japanese breakfast and June the American one (bacon and eggs). Barbara, gleefully chopsticking down the exotic (often unrecognizable) delights, told June, "You're really lucky. You get to eat the breakfast you're used to, but you still get to see my beautiful Japanese breakfast." "Yes," replied June, "and smell it."

In Guadalajara, we ate breakfast *(desayuno)* every morning at a little side-street cafe, La Tupinamba, where we often had tortillas filled with scrambled eggs and spiced up with salsa. Thanks to La Tortilla's low-carb, fat-free tortillas, you can do your own La Tupinamba variation. Yes, it has eggs, but it's a nice change from the standard American classic, and you could always use cheese instead of eggs for a similar effect.

An Italian treat we often have for breakfast is not served for breakfast there, but rather as an appetizer: *insalata caprese*. Start with some mozzarella cheese (small balls of soft, fresh mozzarella if you can find it; slices of a large, firm mozzarella if you can't). Decorate this with a few very thin slices of tomato—very few, very thin, as tomato, really a fruit, is high in carbohydrate. (Dr. Bernstein wouldn't even approve of this small amount.) Sprinkle with fresh basil if you have it, dried if you don't, and lightly drizzle everything with extra-virgin olive oil. A few of those little wrinkled, oil-cured black olives are a nice touch, too.

In the delis of New York and southern California and a growing number of places in between, lox (smoked salmon) and bagels and cream cheese are a breakfast—and brunch—staple. They're becoming a staple for us as well. Without the bagel, of course. Those guys are carbohydrate bombs, with half a bagel ranging from thirty to sixty grams, depending on the size. But nothing is better than some kind of smoked salmon—nova (for Nova Scotia), Norwegian, Scottish (Queen Elizabeth's favorite), Irish, etc.—with cream cheese on a crisp bread. If you're eligible for a bit more carbohydrate, you could add a thin slice of a crisp, sweet onion (red, Maui, or Vidalia). Again, Dr. Bernstein would say, "Tsk, tsk."

Sometimes we stay at hotels that, as part of a special, provide a continental breakfast. One of these breakfasts, at the Four Seasons Biltmore in Santa Barbara, was lavish—it offered all kinds of bread, including croissants and bagels, a fruit plate, and fruit juice. A real carbo-a-thon. We did some quick math and discovered that for the same price as the continental breakfasts, we could share an order of eggs with ham or bacon or sausage, or even Eggs Benedict. We asked if we could make a substitution, and indeed we could.

Dinner for Breakfast

Years ago, talking about traveling across America, we suggested that if none of the cafes in a town where you needed to eat looked too promising, you should order breakfast no matter what time of day it was, because almost any eatery can put together a decent bacon or ham and egg dish. Now we suggest reversing the process: Eat what you normally would for lunch or dinner for breakfast.

We got this idea from Dr. Lois Jovanovic-Peterson, who often puts her pregnant patients on a low-carb, high-protein diet to stabilize their blood sugars. As a wife and mother herself, she knows you don't always have the time to fix the protein food you need, so she suggests eating the left-over protein from the previous night's dinner. For some people the idea of lamb stew or barbecued chicken or meat loaf for breakfast takes a bit of mental adjustment, but once you get used to it, it can be fun and certainly is never dull.

A friend of ours who was a fantastic gourmet cook used to have elaborate dinner parties. The next morning, exhausted from her party activities, she'd feed her junior-high-age son the leftovers. One morning, as he was eating the previous night's fare, he mused, "Gee, Mom, I'll bet I'm the only boy in the San Fernando Valley who's having quail with black grapes and wild rice fritters and Brussels sprouts mousse for breakfast." Since he grew up and went to medical school and continued on to become a psychiatrist, apparently his unorthodox breakfast fare didn't do him any harm—or did it?

P.S. If you—like many of us these days—hardly have time to fix and eat anything, there's always a quick Protein 21 Bar or a protein shake from Take Care.

Eating Out

Actually, eating in restaurants doesn't pose much of a problem. Since most diners are on some kind of specialized diet, restaurants are increasingly willing—and in some cases actually happy—to accommodate you. It shows off their culinary talents and virtuosity. Long before she started the low-carb diet, Barbara used to redesign almost every dish in a restaurant, substituting items that more pleased her fancy for ones that didn't intrigue her. She was in perfect training for making low-carb adjustments. One kind of place where it's difficult if not impossible to get substitutions is at a fast-food dispensary. But then, you shouldn't be there anyway. Chinese restaurants also aren't big on substitutions, but there's usually so much variety on the menu that you can put together an appropriate meal.

Another trick of the low-carb trade is to go for appetizers rather than main courses. Main courses usually come with accompaniments of the high-carb persuasion—the ubiquitous pasta, potatoes, or rice—and even the vegetables run to the root ones, such as carrots, which are very high in carbohydrates. When we do order a main dish we ask for "only green vegetables" with it.

When possible, we also order half portions. This is easier to do in Europe than in this country, but more and more restaurants here are starting this happy trend. By the way, in Italy, where even the most fanatic low-carber is wont to succumb to the delectable pastas, we order a *mezza portione,* also called *uno per due* (one for two), and we split it. If we've walked all morning and then walk all afternoon, we can get away with it. We call this our "We walk for pasta tour of Italy."

Doggie bags, YES! Everybody's doing it these days. It's not chic to waste food. The Ann Landers column in which she said it was "tacky" to take foods home from restaurants yielded her an avalanche of negative mail. One of the letters was from a maitre d' who thought it was a great idea and even considered it a compliment to the restaurant if you want to take home your leftovers. If we've ordered correctly and take food home, we can often make a lovely low-carb lunch the next day.

Emergency rations: A couple of dishes that can be found on many menus are perfect for a low-carber: a chicken Caesar salad or a Cobb salad (contains chicken, hard-boiled egg, bacon, and roquefort, Gorgonzola, or blue cheese).

Fear of Ketones

Some of those who follow the low-carb diet for weight loss worry about the ketones produced in the body by the burning of fat. All of us involved with diabetes have learned to fear ketones as the harbingers of diabetic coma—and worse. But Drs. Ezrin and Eades say that this is only true for out-of-control type 1 diabetics in ketoacidosis. The "mild, beneficial" ketosis of the weight-loss phase of their low-carbohydrate diets is a normal stage of fat breakdown. Read their books for a complete explanation of the science involved. Dr. Bernstein advises type 1's on the diet who (or whose physicians!) are disturbed by even mild ketones to keep testing for them and gradually increase carbohydrate and insulin until they disappear.

ANECDOTAL EVIDENCE IN FAVOR OF THE LOW-CARBOHYDRATE DIET

In diabetes—as in all health conditions—there are two kinds of evidence of how well therapies work. There is scientific evidence, and there is anecdotal evidence. Scientific evidence is universally praised and respected for its accuracy and validity. Anecdotal evidence is scorned as unreliable and invalid, especially by scientists and health professionals. *New York Times* columnist Russell Baker says that by calling something anecdotal evidence scientists suggest it is worthless to listen to mere people. They want all evidence to be "free of odious anecdotal taint."

We always laugh when we see headlines shouting, "Scientific Breakthrough in the Search for a Cure for Diabetes," because we know the "breakthrough" was based on experiments with six mice in New Jersey, and the end of the article admits it will be years before we know if it works for humans.

Anecdotal evidence, on the other hand, we define as "what really happens to real people and they tell you about it." Therefore, we're giving you some anecdotes—we call them "humanecdotes"—on the effectiveness of the low-carb diet. Incidentally, Dean Esmay, free-lance low-carb diet researcher and author of *The World's Biggest Fad Diet (And Why You Should Probably Avoid It)* says, "Individual experiences are not 'anecdotal' if the people have taken the time to get the medical tests and can show empirically that they, personally, are healthy." Most of the following people, as diabetics who monitor all aspects of their health, can empirically show this.

After the publication of *Diabetes Type II and What to Do,* we received a letter from an articulate woman named Ann. It is forever etched on our memories, because it nearly fried our eyeballs. A shortened—and expurgated—version is:

"I'm sick of reading your books in which June is so [expletive deleted] perky about her diabetes and how easy it is to control it. Well I want you to know there is no way this [expletive deleted] disease can be controlled."

Then, about a month after the publication of the issue of *Diabetic Reader* in which we discussed the advantages of the low-carb diet, we received the following fax:

> I know you guys thought you'd never hear from me again, but I had to let you know that I was so glad to read about the low-carb, high-protein diet extolled in the latest issue. This has simply cured my type 2 problem. I tried fat-free and my blood sugar was consistently out of whack, my face looked like I had adolescent acne, and I had no energy and constant heartburn. Once I tried the low-carb diet, I

have found myself again—that incredible, energetic girl I once knew. I am not as hungry, my blood sugar is A-OK, and I am more muscular and stronger. No more heartburn either.

My father has finally stopped his yo-yo dieting with this diet, and my poor mother-in-law, who was diagnosed with type 2 a year ago, is still following the terrible advice given to her by her stupid doctor and remains on the low-fat diet and out of control.

Barbara H. has had type 1 diabetes for eighteen years. She was overweight, and her blood sugars rarely struck the middle ground. It was not unusual for her to hit 350 once a day and drop to 50 or so with an insulin reaction if she wasn't paying attention. Then she started experimenting with a high-protein diet and limited carbs.

My first blood-sugar reading at 6 P.M. on the first day was 103. I don't think I've ever been 103, especially at 6 P.M. My next reading was 97. I was flabbergasted. I don't think I've ever had those readings: maybe 369 or 64, but nothing close to normal. Hello out there, ADA, AMA, and the grain industry. Why didn't someone tell me that low carb/high protein was the way to stabilize and control blood sugar?

Soon I began having low-blood-sugar reactions, so I began reducing my insulin. It became clear that I'd better ease into this slowly and stabilize my insulin dose and forget about losing weight at first. Formerly I took twenty-eight units of NPH in the morning and eight units around 8 P.M. plus two units of Regular to cover meals/overeating. Very often I would take an additional two units at bedtime. Now I'm taking twenty-four units of NPH in the morning and four or five units in the evening and absolutely no Regular, unless I eat a cherry pie or something. My blood sugars stay below 150 and above 90 if I continue to eat protein as my major source of food. This is nothing short of a miracle for me. I am enjoying the entirely new experience of being able to sleep through the night without waking to a high or a low reaction and living through the day relatively free of the needle and holding blood sugar middle ground. Heaven, I'm in heaven.

Fran B. wrote:

> I've just been talking to a friend of my daughter's who is diabetic. She knows a diabetic girl who is a concert violist and diabetic. She was not having much luck in controlling her blood sugar with the typical diet recommended for diabetics. It is especially difficult because she travels extensively. Also being a teenager with galloping hormones doesn't help. Her mother happened to meet a nurse whose son is diabetic, and she said they were having great success [with the low-carb, high-protein diet]. This young girl has been in perfect control for the last four months following this diet. She doesn't seem to be affected by the stress of her profession, at least not in terms of her blood sugar.

From Judy W.:

> I was delighted to see your review of Dr. Calvin Ezrin's new book [*Type 2 Diabetes Diet Book*]. I have personal experience with this diet. At Dr. Ezrin's office today I weighed 146½ pounds, exactly 100 pounds less than when I started his program 434 days ago. When I lose ten to twenty pounds more, I'll be at the weight I reached in 1978, 1969, 1964, and 1957. These valleys were achieved on Weight Watchers, pills, and Slenderella. Each was followed by a new peak. After losing seventy pounds in 1978, I gained 130 pounds between 1980 and 1991. I'm 5′ 5″. My top weight was 260.
>
> This time I've gone from a size 22/24 to a 10/12. I've always saved my thin clothes, because I would buy nice things to celebrate my new figure and then start gaining again and never wear them out. I'm rediscovering a whole new/old wardrobe, and I'm right in (retro) fashion.
>
> Before Dr. Ezrin's program, no matter how much I ate, I would

feel a gnawing emptiness within twenty minutes, and I had virtually given up resisting it. Then my mother developed diabetes, and I realized the risks I was running.

The first miracle Dr. Ezrin's program worked was to wipe out my irresistible craving for carbohydrates. Now I'm only hungry when I'm supposed to be. I don't see myself resuming the way I used to eat when I reach my goal, because now I don't miss carbohydrates. The second miracle was to unleash in me so much energy, positive mood, and healthy body awareness that I began to *want* to exercise.

This time life began at sixty. I've become leaner, stronger, and shapelier, but much more important, I have natural energy, a manageable appetite, and a serenity I've never experienced. For the first time in my life I think I know how normal people feel.

From D.D. on the Internet:

What I found, after ninety days of low-carbing, was that not only was my glycoHgb the best it had been since diagnosis, [but also] my cholesterol stayed the same, and my HDL was MUCH higher, and my LDL lower. . . . Also triglycerides, which had been markedly elevated, were near normal. And I lost twenty pounds in three months, without dieting, over the Christmas holidays. Pretty encouraging, and the best part was my diabetes counselor, who was aghast at my eating plan, was sure I was headed for Doom. She was left sputtering. . . . I also have friends who are managing their diabetes on a high-carb vegetarian plan, and doing well. So we HAVE to leave room for people with those other kinds of metabolisms, who don't handle fats well. Lucky for me, I can still have my cheesecake and eat it too!

I guess our favorite communication has to be the one from an old friend in diabetes, Elsie Smallback, R.N., B.S.N., C.D.E. Elsie worked with us back when we had the SugarFree Centers for Diabetics. We saw her struggle with her weight and cholesterol . . . Well, let her tell the story.

Congratulations. You've done it again. You tested a most controversial diet. And only after remaining on this diet for two years and experiencing remarkably successful results in blood-sugar control, blood chemistry levels, and weight management did you report . . . these findings to your readers. . . . Your write-up made the low-carbohydrate diet credible for me. . . . I tried it. After three months I had my cholesterol tested. I am amazed!! For the past ten years my cholesterol has ranged from a high of 284 to 224 on a low-fat "balanced" diet. My weight steadily climbed up despite daily brisk walks of four to six miles. I felt resigned to the dreaded middle-age spread. No more. Now I can brag a 196 cholesterol and a weight loss of fifteen pounds. And I know six other persons personally who are having the same results.

—Elsie

P.S. Too bad that dietitian who asked to have her name removed from your mailing list doesn't have a more open mind. She might have been able to help more of her patients.

We have more, but these reports give you an idea of how the diet has worked for some people. As of this writing, we've been on the diet for over three years. Will we stay on it forever? We don't know. Actually, the diabetic diet—like life—is more a journey than a destination. Diabetic diets change as knowledge and tools for diabetic control improve, and so, probably, will ours. We always try to follow the advice they give in medical school: "Never be the first—or the last—to try a new therapy." If and when we do try a new diet, we promise to let you know how it works out. And we hope you'll let us know about your dietary adventures. But while you're traveling on your personal diabetic diet journey, we hope you'll remember what our heroine and sometime low-carber Julia Child said in the last line of her first book: "Above all have a good time."

Reference Section

MEDICATIONS THAT INCREASE BLOOD-GLUCOSE LEVELS	MEDICATIONS THAT LOWER BLOOD-GLUCOSE LEVELS
Chlorthalidone	Ethyl alcohol
Corticosteroids	Insulin
Diazoxide	Sulfonylureas
Furosemide	Beta blockers
Epinephrine-like medications	Anabolic steroids
Estrogens	Fenfluramine
Nicotinic acid	Biguanides
Phenytoin	Salicylates (large doses)
Syrups containing sugar	Disopyramide
Thyroid preparations	Phenobarbital (and other enzyme inducers)
Thiazide	
Glucagon	
Caffeine (large quantities)	
Cyclophosphamide	
Ethacrynic acid	
Asparaginase	
Morphine	
Nicotine	
Lithium	

DIRECTORY OF ORGANIZATIONS

American Association of Diabetes Educators
444 N. Michigan Ave., Ste. 1240
Chicago, IL 60601
1-800-338-DMED
Write for information on diabetes education programs and a list of certified diabetes educators in your area.

American Diabetes Association
1660 Duke St.
Alexandria, VA 22314
1-800-ADA-DISC
Write for the address of your local chapter if it is not listed in your phone book.

American Dietetic Association
216 W. Jackson Blvd., Ste. 800
Chicago, IL 60606-6995
1-800-366-1655
Can provide names of qualified dietitians in your area.

International Diabetic Athletes Association
6829 N. 12th St., Ste. 205
Phoenix, AZ 85014
602-230-8155
A nonprofit organization to foster interaction among active individuals with diabetes who participate in sports and fitness activities at all levels, health care professionals, and everyone interested in the relationship between (or special problems of) diabetes and sports.

Juvenile Diabetes Foundation International
120 Wall St., 19th Fl.
New York, NY 10005

1-800-223-1138

A national group whose objective is to fund research aimed at curing diabetes and preventing its complications. Information, educational programs, and meetings for diabetic children and young people and their families. Write for address of your local chapter.

DIABETES WEB SITES

Many of the companies making diabetes equipment and supplies have their own Web sites to give information on their products. You'll usually find these addresses on their ads in diabetes publications and in product inserts.

Web sites are proliferating like fruit flies. If you hack around using the word "diabetes" as your machete, you'll come up with more sites than you'll possibly have time to explore. Just don't take everything you read on the Internet as gospel. Along with the sound and useful information, you'll find some Strange Stuff with little or no basis in reality or concern for scientific accuracy. As in all areas of diabetes self-care, you have to be wise and beware in order to be well.

American Association of Clinical Endocrinologists
http://www.aace.com

American Association of Diabetes Educators
http://www.aadenet.org

American Diabetes Association
http://www.diabetes.org

American Dietetic Association
http://www.eatright.org

Canadian Diabetes Association (in both French and English)
http://www.diabetes.ca/

Emory University Health Sciences Center Library. MedWeb
http://www.cc.emory.edu/WHSCL/medweb.html

Federal Center for Disease Control Diabetes Page
http://www.cdc.gov/nccdphp/ddt/dthome.htm

Juvenile Diabetes Foundation International
http://www.jdfcure.com

LC-Diabetes (A support list for all persons restricting intake of carbohydrates as a method of diabetes management in order to avoid and control diabetic complications)
http://www.mountain-inter.net/~magnuson/

LC-Diabetes Archives
http://maelstrom.stjohns.edu/archives/LC-DIABETES.html

International Diabetic Athletes Association
idaa@getnet.com

Lehigh Diabetic Archives
http://www.lehigh.edu/lists/diabetic/

National Institutes of Health
http://www.niddk.nih.gov/

Ohio State University
http://www.cis.ohio-state.edu/hypertext/faq/usenet/
diabetes/top.html

On-Line Resources for Diabetics
http://gate.cruzio.com/~mendosa/faq.htm

Prana Publications (*Diabetic Reader,* June Biermann & Barbara Toohey)
http://members.aol.com/prana2

Reuters Health Information Services, Inc.
http://www.reutershealth.com/news

University of Miami Diabetes Research International Network (Drinet)
http://drinet.med.miami.edu

University of Wisconsin Diabetes Knowledgebase
http://www.biostat.wisc.edu/diaknow.index.htm

HOW SWEET IT IS

Aspartame	A protein sweetener 180 times as sweet as sucrose. Technically, aspartame is caloric; however, it is so sweet that the amount used per serving of food is likely to supply almost no calories. Marketed as Equal and NutraSweet.
Carob Powder Carob flour	Produced by grinding the pod of the carob tree. Tastes similar to chocolate. Seventy-five percent is made up of sucrose, glucose, and fructose, which are all caloric.
*Cyclamates**	*Noncaloric* sweeteners approximately thirty times as sweet as sucrose. Cyclamates were banned from use in the United States in 1970 because of questions about their possible cancer- and tumor-causing properties. They are still used in some foreign countries, and the risk associated with moderate use is considered by many to be very small. In 1989 it was announced that the U.S. ban on cyclamates would be lifted, but this has not happened.
Dextrin	Chains of glucose molecules. Their effect on blood glucose has not been well evaluated but may be similar to glucose. Caloric.
Dulcitol	A sugar alcohol. Caloric.
Fructose Fruit sugar Levulose	One of the most common naturally occurring sugars, particularly found in fruit and honey. It is not associated with a rapid and high rise in blood sugar in well-

*The sweeteners in italics are generally felt to be appropriate sweeteners for the diabetic individual, provided they are used according to the recommendation of a physician or dietitian.

controlled diabetes. The sweetness of refined fructose varies, but under certain conditions it can be almost twice as sweet as sucrose. Caloric.

Glucose
Corn sugar
Dextrose
Grape sugar

A naturally occurring sugar that normally causes a fast and high rise in blood sugar. About half as sweet as table sugar. Carbohydrates (starches) break down to glucose during digestion, as do all sugars eventually. Glucose is the form of sugar that the body uses for energy and other purposes, and it builds up in the blood if diabetes is poorly controlled. *Dextrose* is the commercial name for glucose and will often be seen on food labels, including those of some sugar substitutes. Caloric.

Glucose Syrups
Corn syrup
Corn-syrup
solids
Sorghum syrup
Starch syrup
Sugar-cane
syrup

Liquid sweeteners produced by the breakdown (hydrolyzation) of starch. They contain a mixture of glucose, maltose, and longer chains of glucose molecules and can be produced from a variety of starches (hence the varied names). *Corn-syrup solids* are the crystallized form of corn syrup. Caloric.

High-Fructose
Corn Syrups

Produced from corn syrups. They contain differing amounts of fructose, ranging from 42 to 90 percent. The remaining part of the syrup is primarily glucose. The effect of the highly refined type (90 percent fructose) on blood glucose has not been well evaluated, but, theoretically, it should not cause high and fast rises of glucose in the blood of people whose diabetes is well controlled. The 90 percent type is the only one that might prove to be an acceptable sweetener for diabetics. Caloric.

Honey Comb honey Creamed honey	A natural syrup that varies in sugar and flavor depending on many factors. It is primarily glucose (about 35 percent), fructose (about 40 percent), and water and, by weight, is about 75 percent as sweet as sucrose. Additional glucose is sometimes added to some honeys. Caloric.
Lactose	Milk sugar. It comprises about 4.5 percent of cow milk. About 30 percent as sweet as sucrose. Caloric.
Maltose	Two glucose units linked together. It is only 30 to 50 percent as sweet as sucrose, but it rapidly breaks down to glucose in the intestinal tract. Caloric.
Mannitol	A naturally occurring sugar alcohol that causes less of a rise in blood sugar than do sucrose or glucose. It is about half as sweet as sucrose and is slowly absorbed into the blood. In large amounts, it can cause diarrhea. Caloric.
Maple Syrup Maple sugar	Made from the sap of the maple and other trees. It is mostly sucrose, with some invert sugar (see *sucrose*) and trace amounts of other compounds. The crystallized syrup is *maple sugar.* Caloric.
Milk Chocolate Bittersweet chocolate	Produced by the addition of milk, sugar, and cocoa butter to bitter chocolate. *Milk chocolate* is approximately 43 percent sugar and *bittersweet chocolate* is about 40 percent sugar. The sugar is caloric.
Molasses Blackstrap Golden syrup Refiners' syrup	The sugar drawn from sugar crystals as they are refined into pure sucrose. Different types are usually produced during sucrose refinement. All types, however, contain 50 to 75 percent sugar (sucrose and in-

Treacle Unsulphured	vert sugar) and should generally be avoided by diabetics. The sugars are caloric.
Saccharin	The currently used *noncaloric* sweetener in the United States. It is about 375 times as sweet as sucrose.
Sorbitol	A naturally occurring sugar alcohol found in many plants; commercially produced from glucose. It is about half as sweet and more slowly absorbed than glucose. In individuals whose diabetes is well controlled, it causes only a small post-meal rise in blood glucose. In large amounts it may cause diarrhea. It is widely used in the manufacture of dietetic foods and chewing gums. Caloric.

Sucrose
  Beet sugar
  Brown sugar
  Cane sugar
  Confectioner's
    sugar
  Invert sugar
  Powdered sugar
  Raw sugar
  Saccharose
  Sugar
  Table sugar
  Turbinado
	A naturally occurring sugar that is composed of equal parts of glucose and fructose linked together. It is produced from sugar cane or sugar beets. *Invert sugar* is made of sucrose that has been broken down to equal parts of glucose and fructose (with some sucrose left intact). *Brown sugars, raw sugar,* and *Turbinado* all contain some molasses.

Sweetened Condensed whole milk	Produced by reducing the water content of milk by about half and adding sugar. The finished product is about 44 percent sucrose, which is caloric. This means a fourteen-ounce can of condensed whole milk con-

Sweetened condensed skim milk Sweetened condensed whey	tains the equivalent of eight tablespoons of sugar and two and a half cups of milk.
Xylitol	A naturally occurring sugar alcohol produced from xylose (bark sugar). It is slowly absorbed and causes less of a rise in blood sugar than does sucrose or glucose. Depending on how it is used, it is as sweet as or less sweet than sucrose. It is believed to be less cavity inducing than other sugars. Large amounts can cause diarrhea, and questions about its safety have held up its use in all but a few products. Caloric.

Courtesy of Phyllis Crapo, R.D., and Margaret A. Powers, R.D., *Diabetes Forecast,* March–April 1981, p. 24. Copyright 1980 by the American Diabetes Association. Reprinted from *Diabetes Forecast* with permission.

DOCTOR'S INITIAL EXAMINATION

On your first visit to a new doctor or shortly thereafter, you should undergo a comprehensive evaluation of your diabetes. The following components are an indispensable part of that evaluation.

COMPLETE HISTORY AND PHYSICAL EXAMINATION

Although the history is probably the most important feature of the initial evaluation, full details cannot be provided here for space reasons. Essential points that should be covered include family history of diabetes; circumstances at the onset of the diabetes; history of treatment through diet, exercise, pills, and insulin; and evaluation of the effectiveness of current treatment. In addition, the presence of or potential for diabetic complications should also be reviewed. These complications are macrovascular (arteriosclerosis affecting circulation to the heart, legs, and brain); microvascular (affecting the retina and kidney); and neuropathic (leading to numbness in the feet, impotence, or other symptoms).

The physical exam should be as comprehensive as any you've ever had. Important aspects of the exam include:

- *Blood pressure.* A risk factor for diabetic complications and a reflection of subtle changes in kidney function.
- *Eyes.* Retinal exam to check for diabetic retinopathy.
- *Neck.* Evaluation for autoimmune thyroid disease.
- *Heart.* Check for macrovascular complications (arteriosclerosis) affecting circulation to the heart.
- *Pulse.* Evaluation for arteriosclerosis. Pulse should be checked in the neck, wrists, groin, top of foot, and inner ankle.
- *Neurological.* Check for sensations in the feet. "Reflexes" checked with a hammer tap at the ankle and knee.

- *Feet.* Examination for pulse and neurological function as well as deformities such as bunions or hammer toes, calluses, breaks in the skin, and improperly cut toenails.

LABORATORY EVALUATION

The following tests are especially important in evaluating a patient with diabetes:

- *Blood sugar.* A seemingly indispensable part of diabetes care, but is *one* blood sugar value really that important, compared with what the patient can test at home?
- *Glycosylated hemoglobin.* Essential in evaluating overall diabetes control and as a baseline for further improvements in therapy.
- *Cholesterol, HDL cholesterol, triglycerides.* Total cholesterol and LDL cholesterol (calculated from the three lipid tests) are used to evaluate the risk of diabetic macrovascular complications. Triglyceride values (which are often elevated in diabetes) may also reflect the level of overall diabetes control.
- *Creatinine.* A measure of kidney function, not especially sensitive to early changes. Measuring "creatinine clearance" by obtaining both a blood test and a twenty-four-hour urine specimen is much more sensitive.
- *Urinalysis.* Important as a screen for infection and to look for urine protein.
- *Microalbuminuria.* The most sensitive measure for early diabetes kidney effect, this test should become the standard for patients with diabetes. It can be measured with a random, overnight, or twenty-four-hour urine collection.
- *Urine culture.* Should be done if the urinalysis shows any abnormality.
- *Thyroid function tests.* Essential for every patient with type 1 diabetes to be screened for autoimmune thyroid disease.

- *Electrocardiogram (EKG)*. Should be done routinely in patients who are over forty or who have had at least ten years of diabetes. A baseline reading is often done on all patients at the first visit.

These data form the basis of your initial evaluation and, in a shortened version, may become the model for a yearly diabetes update. But remember—medical care cannot be evaluated by a checklist; your own physician may have a different way of organizing the above data. Still, one way or another, this information should be part of every diabetic patient's record. Knowing what to expect, and what data to ask for, will help you become more informed about your own health and medical care.

RECOMMENDED READING AND LISTENING

Note: The following books are available at most major bookstores or from Prana Publications, 5623 Matilija Ave., Van Nuys, CA 91401 (call 1-800-735-7726 for information). The audio tapes are also available from Prana Publications.

BOOKS FOR EVERYONE

Black Health Library Guide to Diabetes, by Lester Henry, Jr., M.D., with Kirk A. Johnson. (1993) 181 pp.

A guide written expressly for African Americans, of whom one in ten has diabetes. By the chief of endocrinology at Howard University, a man with more than fifty years' experience treating diabetes. His book tells people what they need to know to respect and survive it. A sound, realistic book, very clearly written, and with a wonderful philosophy.

Diabetes: A Practical New Guide to Healthy Living, by James Anderson, M.D. (1981) 210 pp.

Dr. Anderson, professor of medicine and clinical nutrition at the University of Kentucky, believes diabetics can lead rewarding lives through proper diet and exercise. Features his High Carbohydrate-Fiber, Low-Fat Nutrition Plan (HCF), which he began developing in 1974. Particularly helpful for overweight, non-insulin-dependent diabetics.

Diabetes A to Z, by the American Diabetes Association (Rev. 1996) 200 pp.

Tells "What You Need to Know About Diabetes: SIMPLY PUT." Alphabetized for quick reference to over fifty important topics, like food labeling, glycohemoglobin tests, exercise, dental care, blood-glucose self-tests, etc.

Diabetes Care Made Easy, by Allison Nemanic, R.N., B.A., and others. (1992) 154 pp.

A step-by-step guide for controlling diabetes. It is written for both children (six- to nine-year olds) and adults and is *extremely* easy to read, with many illustrations that make for clear understanding. Covers all the basics: taking insulin, what to eat, exercises, testing blood sugar, coping with emotions.

Diabetes Is Not a Piece of Cake, by Janet Meirelles, R.N., C.D.E. (1994) 288 pp.

Full of information and empathy for the long-ignored nondiabetic who shares life with a person with diabetes. Opens lines of communication, smooths out conflicts, and improves the relationship and eases the burden on both sides. Clearly written; based on three hundred questionnaires and Janet's professional experience. The reference section is full of timely where-to-find-it and how-to-handle-it information.

Diabetes Mellitus: A Practical Handbook, by Sue K. Milchovich, R.N., C.D.E., and Barbara Dunn-Long, R.D. (6th rev. ed. 1995) 200 pp.

An easy-to-use and thorough explanation of diabetes and how to control it. Very complete on diet and food choices (includes the entire set of Exchange Lists); has sample meal plans for different calorie levels. Large type. Excellent for beginners.

Diabetes Sourcebook, by Diana Guthrie, R.N., Ph.D., and Richard Guthrie, M.D. (3rd ed. 1997) 286 pp.

Subtitled *Today's Methods and Ways to Give Yourself the Best Care,* this basic book is distinctive because the Guthries, whom we have known since 1979, have always been at the forefront of diabetes therapy and education. Trust them implicitly to help you in every daily aspect of diabetes care. It's all here, from testing equipment to stress management, to food guides, to family support, to working with your doctor, to dental care, to sex, to exercise.

The Diabetic Man, by Peter A. Lodewick, M.D., June Biermann, and Barbara Toohey. (Updated ed. 1996) 348 pp.

The guide to health and success in all areas of a man's life: career, sports, travel, sex, and relationships. Includes advice, empathy, and support for those with a diabetic man in their lives and for parents of a diabetic son. Dr. Lodewick is an endocrinologist, a sportsman, and a well-controlled diabetic.

The Diabetic Woman, by Lois Jovanovic-Peterson, M.D., June Biermann, and Barbara Toohey. (Rev. 1996) 286 pp.

The only book that tells how women can deal with diabetes-related problems at different life stages. Medical advice and realistic coping methods for the complex concerns of today's woman. Supplements on type 1 pregnancy and gestational pregnancy. Dr. Jovanovic-Peterson is an endocrinologist specializing in the problems of diabetic women, a senior scientist at Sansum Medical Research Foundation in Santa Barbara, a diabetic, a wife, a mother, and, as this book shows, a warm, caring person.

The Diabetic's Total Health Book, by June Biermann and Barbara Toohey. (3rd ed. 1992) 302 pp.

The book that proves you can have diabetes yet be the picture of health, leading a vital, productive, happy life. How to focus on health rather than on disease and how to achieve a strong body, a tranquil mind, and a blithe spirit. Entertaining—and effective!—sections on reducing stress and raising your spirits with travel, laughter, and hugs. Besides the latest in diabetes therapy, there are sections on weight training for all ages, growing your own vegetables with no-work gardening, and thirty-five of June and Barbara's favorite recipes.

How to Get Great Diabetes Care, by Irl B. Hirsch, M.D. (1996) 180 pp.

This invaluable manual is a first-of-its-kind. Its title describes perfectly exactly how it will help you. It tells you the best standards of care and explains what you need to know to demand them of your doctors, nurses, and HMO.

The Joslin Guide to Diabetes: A Program for Managing Your Treatment, by Richard S. Beaser, M.D., with Joan V.C. Hill, R.D., C.D.E. (1995) 351 pp.

How to give yourself the best possible treatment. Describes the therapeutic options open to you to avoid the negative consequences of outmoded and bad therapy. What and when to eat, monitoring blood sugars, administering insulin and oral medications, treating high and low blood sugars, plus sections on exercise, children with diabetes, pregnancy, sexual issues, etc. Many charts.

The Johns Hopkins Guide to Diabetes, by Christopher D. Saudek, M.D., Richard R. Rubin, Ph.D., C.D.E., and Cynthia S. Shump, R.D., C.D.E. (1997) 422 pp.

By three professionals from the respected Johns Hopkins University Diabetes Center, this new comprehensive home reference guide is absolutely authoritative and up to date. Its unique emphasis is to bring you, the patient, into the picture and to address all your concerns—medical, financial, and emotional. Everything you need to know for good control, good health, and a good life. Over thirty-four illustrations.

Living with Diabetic Complications, by Judy Curtis. (1993) 294 pp.

A book by and for people who live with serious diabetic complications. Never dismal, whiny, or preachy, it's supportive, informative, and positive. Sound, workable strategies for coping physically and emotionally. Thorough and competent guidance on medical treatment options plus sources of additional specialized help. Judy, diabetic for forty-two years, has experienced vision impairment, kidney and heart disease, neuropathy, and an amputation. She's a perfect role model and an honest and caring writer. Incorporates answers to questionnaires sent to hundreds of people with complications. A one-of-a-kind book.

Managing Diabetes on a Budget, by Leslie Y. Dawson. American Diabetes Association. (1995) 90 pp.

Tips and hints on how to get value for every dollar you spend on diabetes self-care. Tells how to comparison-shop for medications and supplies, shop smart for groceries, get the most out of your insurance coverage, and even how to avoid complications.

101 Tips for Staying Healthy with Diabetes, by the University of New Mexico Diabetes Care Group. (1996) 112 pp.

The inside track on easy-to-follow techniques for preventing and treating complications. Question and answer format. Sample subjects: reducing pain of finger sticks, treating and preventing skin infections, avoiding inappropriate flu and cold medicines, etc.

Reversing Diabetes, by Julian Whitaker, M.D. (1987) 389 pp.

Dr. Whitaker, inspired by the writings of Nathan Pritikin, has long championed a life-style program for diabetics and heart patients based on diet and exercise. At his Wellness Institute in Newport Beach, California, he's treated thousands of patients with his system of a diet high in complex carbohydrates and fiber and a program of exercise four to six days per week. He also advocates vitamin and mineral supplements. This book provides the rationale for a high-carbohydrate, low-fat diet and includes a month of menus with over one hundred recipes. A complete do-it-by-the-book program.

FOR SPANISH SPEAKERS

La Diabetes y el Cuidado Fácil, por Allison Nemic, R.N., B.A., y otros. (1992) 154 pp.

This step-by-step guide for controlling diabetes is written for both children and adults. Very easy to read with many illustrations that make for clear understanding.

FOR PEOPLE TAKING INSULIN

Diabetes 101, by Betty Page Brackenridge, M.S., R.D., C.D.E., and Richard O. Dolinar, M.D. (Rev. 2nd ed. 1993) 208 pp.

A diabetes survival guide answering the questions faced by all insulin takers. Told in true-life stories that are engaging and fun to read. No medical jargon. Includes every aspect of self-care to help you control your diabetes and your life. If the idea of going onto insulin makes your hair stand on end, reading this will make your hair—and all the rest of you—relax.

The Diabetes Self-Care Method, by Charles Peterson, M.D., and Lois Jovanovic-Peterson, M.D. (1990) 154 pp.

An innovative, successful program by two of the foremost endocrinologists of the United States. (Dr. Jovanovic-Peterson is diabetic.) Focuses on normalizing blood sugar through self-testing and insulin adjustment to give you a free and flexible life-style. Exactly the kind of self-care the DCCT recommends for avoiding complications.

The Pocket Pancreas: My Other Checkbook, by John Walsh, P.A., C.D.E., and Ruth Roberts, M.A. (1994) 44 pp.

Whether you use one shot a day, multiple injections, or a pump, this mighty midget of a checkbook-size reference is extremely handy. Contains an amazing amount of concise information to help balance your insulin, food, and exercise most effectively. Includes insulin (types, multiple injections, sensitivity, meal timing), carbohydrate counting (carbohydrate values of most basic foods and grams of carbohydrate used per hour in different exercises), handling low and high blood sugars, and the Carbohydrate Glycemic Index.

Stop the Rollercoaster, by John Walsh, P.A., C.D.E., Ruth Roberts, and Lois Jovanovic-Peterson, M.D. (1995) 192 pp.

If you have inexplicable blood-sugar climbs and plunges, here's help. Written by three highly experienced professionals—two with insulin-dependent diabetes—it introduces Flexible Insulin Therapy, their proven-successful method of using multiple injections to mimic the body's way of maintaining normal blood sugar to give you a flexible life-style and a complication-free future. How to match doses to food and exercise, adjust for highs, lows and emergencies, chart blood sugars, and handle costs. Includes charts, graphs, and formulas for individualization of self-care.

AUDIO CASSETTES

Getting Started with Humalog, by Betty Brackenridge, R.D., M.S., C.D.E., and Kris Swenson, R.N., C.D.E. (1997) 90 min.

Humalog is a new fast-acting insulin every insulin user should know about in order to decide if it might help blood-sugar control. The authors were involved in the clinical trials for FDA approval. This step-by-step guide tells who is likely to benefit from Humalog, how to get started, and how to coordinate with food. Reports of actual patient cases. Special tips such as wherever you inject it, it absorbs at the same rate; eating too much fiber slows down digestion of carbohydrate and may cause a problem. Also covers children, pregnancy, and the pump. Accompanied by useful pamphlet material.

FOR THOSE FOLLOWING
THE LOW-CARBOHYDRATE DIET

See also *Type 2 Diabetes, Weight Loss,* and *Cookbooks: Low Carbohydrate.*

Dr. Bernstein's Diabetes Solution: A Complete Guide to Achieving Normal Blood Sugars, by Richard Bernstein, M.D. (1997) 400 pp.

During the twenty years we've known him, Dr. Bernstein has

come up with one original idea after another, almost always sticking his neck out against prevailing medical opinion.

His plan limits carbohydrate to thirty grams daily, divided 6-12-12 for the three meals. He insists on a blood-sugar goal of 85–90, the same as nondiabetics have. Along with clear, detailed instructions on how to handle virtually every aspect of caring for types 1 and 2 diabetes, he reveals several surprise benefits such as increased alertness, relief from chronic tiredness, improved short-term memory, a new sense of well-being, and the wonderful feeling that we're not doomed to disabling complications and premature death.

Dr. Atkins' New Diet Revolution, by Robert C. Atkins, M.D. (1992) 329 pp.

Dr. Atkins believes a disturbed carbohydrate mechanism is responsible for obesity in 95 percent of people. He calls insulin the hormone that makes you fat and blames insulin resistance and hyperinsulinism for the health problems obesity creates, including diabetes. His diet changes the metabolism to correct this condition. The initial fourteen-day weight-loss diet limits you to twenty grams of carbohydrate daily, but the maintenance allows twenty-five to ninety grams. He asks, "On what level of carbohydrate do you feel the best?" Blood-sugar control levels in diabetes are up to you, as is the exact diet you end up on. You're the one who personalizes and executes the diet. Includes carbo-counting charts and sixty-six recipes that are especially good; he cautions that some are high in fat and to be used only as special treats.

Protein Power, by Michael Eades, M.D., and Mary Dan Eades, M.D. (1996) 338 pp.

This eye-opening, scientifically convincing low-carbohydrate diet book describes how this dietary approach manages obesity, type 2 diabetes, heart disease, high blood pressure, and elevated cholesterol. A wonderfully complete manual explaining that the diet works by restricting carbohydrate to reduce the body's insulin production. Detailed instructions and formulas for designing your own meals with adequate protein, carbohydrate, fiber, and "good" fats. Includes meal plans, a mini-cookbook, snack foods, and vitamin and mineral supplements. A reliable guide to all you need to know and do for success in weight and blood-sugar control for Type 2's, with much useful information for Type 1's.

The Type II Diabetes Diet Book, by Calvin Ezrin, M.D., and Robert E. Kowalski. (Updated ed. 1997) 304 pp.

Dr. Ezrin, an eminent endocrinologist, is one of the pioneers in using a low-carbohydrate diet for weight loss. His new book is directed to type 2's who are at least 20 percent overweight. His research and clinical experience have taught him that such people suffer from an identifiable hormonal disorder called hyperinsulinism. His Insulin Control Diet is a way to reverse hyperinsulinism so that the body can switch gears and start to burn excess fat as fuel. The diet ensures weight loss of up to three pounds for women and four pounds for men per week "without much hunger at all." Only forty grams of carbohydrate are allowed daily, but fifty to seventy-five grams of protein are included, and fat is restricted. Suggested in combination with the diet is a nonintimidating exercise plan and relaxation techniques. Includes meal plans, food charts, and recipes, plus guidance on switching to a stabilization phase.

The World's Biggest Fad Diet (And Why You Should Probably Avoid It), by Dean Esmay. (1997) 12 pp.

Here's a switch. The "fad diet" is not the low-carb one, as you would expect, but rather the low-fat diet. Here Esmay explores "the extraordinarily widespread belief that excessive fat in the diet is the primary cause of obesity, heart disease, and other health problems." He cites and summarizes articles from some of the world's most prestigious medical journals that give evidence that low-fat diets are by and large ineffective and possibly even dangerous. Esmay is a passionate and thorough researcher who has amassed a startling amount of evidence. Also included is his personal journey of discovery on the low-carb diet.

AUDIO CASSETTES

The Bernstein Plan: Types I and II, by Richard K. Bernstein, M.D. (1995)

Type 1: Dr. Bernstein clearly explains his good control regimen: the low-carbohydrate diet, muscle-building through anaerobic exercise, multiple blood-sugar tests, multiple small doses of insulin, how to prevent hypoglycemia, sick days, and understanding gastroparesis. (Two tapes, 90 min. each.)

Type 2: Same principles as type 1. If medication is needed, metformin is used. (If you take insulin, use the type 1 tapes.) How to break the obesity cycle by cutting carbohydrates to reduce hunger, normalize blood sugar, and lose weight. Reducing insulin resistance by building lean body mass. (Two tapes, 90 min. each.)

The Low Carbohydrate Diet for Type II Diabetes, by Linda Sherman, R.D., Psy.D. (1996) 45 min.

A basic introduction to a non-extreme low-carbohydrate diet for weight loss, blood-sugar control, and other health benefits. Dietitian Linda Sherman, who works with Dr. Judith Reichman of Cedars Sinai Medical Center in Los Angeles, has taught this eating plan for fifteen years and uses it herself. Linda clearly explains what to eat, when, and why in the three stages of the diet: (1) weight loss; (2) stabilization; and (3) maintenance. This plan allows for total individualization. A sample of a typical day of meals clarifies the concept and gives you a true taste of this eating style. A simple written guide accompanies the tape.

INSULIN PUMPS

The Insulin Pump Therapy Book, edited by Linda Fredrickson, M.A., R.N., C.D.E. (1995) 160 pp.

If you're on an insulin pump or thinking about one, this book of

"Insights from the Experts" is vital! From the professional education department of MiniMed Technologies, it's a phenomenal reference loaded with the most timely and sophisticated information. Eighteen leading experts with well-deserved worldwide reputations tell you what they know about setting insulin dosages, preventing hypoglycemia, exercise and insulin adjustment, carbohydrate counting, and pregnancy.

Pumping Insulin, by John Walsh, P.A., C.D.E., and Ruth Roberts, M.S. (2nd rev. ed. 1994) 156 pp.

Many people in the Diabetes Control and Complications Trial, which proved the benefits of tight control, used a pump instead of syringes for their insulin. Written by a ten-year veteran pump user, this new second edition of the classic book gives you all the information you need for deciding whether or not to go onto a pump and all the tools you need for the successful use of one.

TYPE 2 DIABETES

See also *Low-Carbohydrate Diet* and *Weight Loss.*

Diabetes Type II and What to Do, by Virginia Valentine, R.N., C.D.E., June Biermann, and Barbara Toohey. (1993) 172 pp.

Nurse-educator Valentine, herself a type 2, gives plain English explanations of the type 2 condition along with advice on how to feel better mentally and physically. She takes the guilt out of having the disease ("It's not a character flaw!") and leads you competently and compassionately into good control. This winner of the AADE's "Educator of the Year" award has a special talent for making anything difficult into something easy and lightening your way to the mastery of good diabetes self-care. Includes Virginia's much-reprinted Gospel, "The Fifteen Commandments for Living Well with Diabetes."

Managing Type II Diabetes, by Arlene Monk, R.D., C.D.E., and others. (Rev., updated 1996) 184 pp.

A mine of the latest therapies and strategies for living with type 2 diabetes. Understandable and encouraging. Explains "routine maintenance" and makes you a genuine partner with the professionals who help you. Has such innovative illustrations as an Activity Pyramid for the exercise aspect of self-care. Excellent survey of all medications and especially helpful blood-glucose-testing tips. Not just a revised edition, but an entirely new book reflecting the latest advances from the staff of the International Diabetes Center in Minneapolis.

WEIGHT LOSS

See also *Low-Carbohydrate Diet and Type 2 Diabetes.*

The Fit or Fat Woman, by Covert Bailey and Lea Bishop. (1989) 151 pp.

Coauthored with biologist and nutrition counselor Lea Bishop, this book applies Covert Bailey's successful weight-loss strategy (see the following entry) to women, acknowledging that "women have more trouble with fat than men." The focus of this program is to lower your body's percentage of fat and increase its percentage of muscle. This requires about sixteen months of daily aerobics and a low-fat, low-sugar diet. Special sections on depression, PMS, anorexia, and bulimia. The science is right up to date, and the fitness advice works and feels good.

The New Fit or Fat?, by Covert Bailey. (Rev. 1991) 167 pp.

The essential message of this well-researched, breakthrough book is that overweight people should concentrate on losing body fat, not pounds. Bailey says that fat people often eat less than skinny people, and the only way they can lose body fat is through exercise that changes their metabolism to burn more fat. "The ultimate cure for obesity is exercise."

Weight Management for Type II Diabetes, by Jackie Labat, M.S., R.D., and Annette Maggi, M.S., R.D. (1997) 176 pp.

Combines nutrition and exercise in a weight control book specifically for type 2 diabetics. Covers setting reasonable exercise goals, keeping pace with an exercise regimen, learning to deal with lapses, developing life-style habits that last, managing stress, teaming up with others for support, and handling special occasions. Includes an "enlightened shopping tour" and a low-fat cooking lesson. Emphasis on taking action yourself, with quizzes and worksheets for you to create your own weight-management success story.

DIABETES AND YOUR EMOTIONS

Diabetes: Caring for Your Emotions as Well as Your Health, by Jerry Edelwich, M.S.W., and Archie Brodsky. (1986) 276 pp.

This is about the *experience* of diabetes and the "inner drama" of people who suffer from it. Uses the actual words and experiences of diabetic people to bring out into the open the feelings that go with having diabetes. Covers a great range of emotional reactions and dilemmas engendered by living with diabetes. Distinguishes between the unique problems of those with type 1 and type 2 diabetes as well as their many common grounds. Excellent on doctors, nurses, family relationships, and support groups.

Psyching Out Diabetes, by Richard R. Rubin, Ph.D., June Biermann, and Barbara Toohey. (Updated 1997) 384 pp.

We've come to believe that diabetes control is 90 percent in your head! This exciting book is a positive guide to your negative emotions that helps you straighten out your head and get rid of the fear, denial, depression, grief, frustration, embarrassment, and guilt that block good diabetes control and a good life. If you're used to seeing diabetes as an enemy, something that complicates your already-too-complex life, this book will show you how to improve your perspective, giving you seven specific frames that will enable you to look at your diabetic challenges in a completely different way. Dr. Rubin, a certified mental health counselor on the faculty of the Johns Hopkins Medical School and in private practice in Baltimore, Maryland, has been counseling diabetic patients for over twenty years. Because he has a diabetic son and a diabetic sister, he has lived with diabetes and knows whereof he speaks—and he speaks clearly, directly, and without any psychological mumbo jumbo.

Reflections on Diabetes, by the American Diabetes Association. (1996) 104 pp.

You may see your own reflection in this collection of personal essays written by people with diabetes who want to share with others their personal experiences with diabetes, relating high moments and low moments and giving their insights and philosophies of overcoming and enduring. All were published in the *Diabetes Forecast* magazine. Learn from others and gain more equilibrium yourself. Perfect for use with support groups and diabetes classes.

AUDIO CASSETTES

Good Times Therapy, by June Biermann and Barbara Toohey (1994) 60 min.

Do you feel that life after diabetes is a drag and a downer? Then you need a shot of "Good Times Therapy." This is not some far-out California idea; it is based on the latest research by psychologists who've discovered that pleasure and the optimism it creates improve your immune system and extend your life. Recorded before a live audience, this tape helps you turn off negative forces and turn on joy; it even shows how diabetes can actually become the key to realizing your life's dreams.

Psyching Out Diabetes, by Richard R. Rubin, Ph.D. (1994) 90 min.

No one speaks more informatively or entertainingly about "Dia-

betes Overwhelmus"—the emotional battle fatigue of all diabetics—
than master storyteller Dr. Richard Rubin, our collaborator on *Psyching Out Diabetes*. He speaks from his thirty-eight years of personal
experience with his diabetic sister and son and his eighteen years of diabetes counseling.

Dr. Rubin makes you feel mentally refreshed and more positive
about diabetes than you ever thought possible.

SPORTS AND EXERCISE

Diabetes Sports and Exercise Book, by Claudia Graham, Ph.D.,
C.D.E., June Biermann, and Barbara Toohey. (1995) 208 pp.

This is a totally new, updated version of our popular 1977 book,
which was based on the sports experiences of 168 diabetic exercise en-
thusiasts. They were the only people who could give help and counsel
at that time, since medical science did not recognize the importance of
exercise for diabetes control and well-being. This 1995 edition contains
all the new scientific and technical information about exercising with
diabetes and teaches you how to attain the marvelous therapeutic effect
of exercise along with all the fun it brings into your life.

Claudia Graham has a Ph.D. in exercise science and is a diabetic
who enthusiastically practices sports. She tells you exactly how to use
sports to the best advantage and how to avoid any possible negative out-
comes. There are special chapters for children, those with complications, and older diabetics.

Diabetes: Your Complete Exercise Guide, by Neil F. Gordon,
M.D., Ph.D., M.P.H. (1993) 137 pp.

Exercise plus diet are the prime therapies for diabetes. There are
scores of food books but fewer than half a dozen exercise books for people with diabetes. What a crazy imbalance! That's why we love this authoritative guide from the famous Cooper Aerobics Center in Dallas.
Tells the real physical payoffs from exercise, how to begin a program,

and how to stick with it. Comprehensive, state-of-the-art advice for both type 1's and type 2's.

The Fitness Book, by the American Diabetes Association. (1995) 149 pp.

Fitness is a necessary goal of all people with diabetes. Claudia Graham, who wrote the chapter on "special needs," defines fitness as "the capacity to meet successfully the present and potential challenges of life." A fitness program has three main elements: stretching, aerobic activity, and muscle strengthening. *The Fitness Book* covers each of them to coach you into shape without undue sweat or tears.

PREGNANCY, DIABETIC CHILD CARE,
AND FAMILY LIFE

Managing your Gestational Diabetes, by Lois Jovanovic-Peterson, M.D., with Morton B. Stone. (1994). 132 pp.

Dr. Jovanovic-Peterson is one of the country's leading authorities on gestational diabetes (a temporary form of diabetes that appears during pregnancy). This book guides you through the steps to control your diabetes and reduce risks to yourself and your baby. Essential reading for mothers-to-be who develop this form of diabetes.

Managing Your Child's Diabetes, by Robert Wood Johnson IV, Sale Johnson, Casey Johnson, and Susan Kleinman. Foreword by Mary Tyler Moore. (Rev. 1996) 199 pp.

Written by a father, mother, and diabetic daughter, this book is vital for parents of newly diagnosed children. The chapter by Casey, diagnosed at the age of eight, is a masterpiece of advice to all parents. The book has detailed information on blood-sugar control (insulin, blood-sugar testing, diet, exercise) as well as dealing with hospitals, teachers, and school.

Parenting a Diabetic Child, by Gloria Loring. (1991) 175 pp.

Singer and actress Gloria Loring is the Celebrity Chairman of the Juvenile Diabetes Foundation. She has parented her diabetic son for over twelve years, so she knows that being a parent is a complex job requiring expert technical information, psychological insight, and emotional support. Gloria provides parents with all three, leading you through the ordeal gently and authoritatively, as only a mother who's been there can.

Sweet Kids, by Betty Brackenridge, M.S., R.D., C.D.E., and Richard R. Rubin, Ph.D., C.D.E. (1996) 314 pp.

Two experienced professionals explain all the intricacies of balancing "diabetes control and good nutrition with family peace." Parents, we assure you that reading *Sweet Kids* will give you both know-how and confidence, and, moreover, you'll delight in its humor and inspiration.

AUDIO CASSETTES

Happy, Healthy Babies: Type 1 Mothers: Gestational, by Lois Jovanovic-Peterson, M.D. (1995) 50 min.

Dr. Jovanovic-Peterson is an eminent endocrinologist who has given medical care to over five hundred pregnant women. She is also a diabetic mother herself and, as you will hear loud and clear on the tape, a warm and compassionate human being. In this audio house call, you can experience all her intelligence, knowledge, experience, and love as she tells you everything you need to know to give birth to a happy, healthy baby: includes medical tests, blood-sugar levels, insulin doses, matching insulin with food, baby testing, labor, delivery, and breast-feeding.

For women who develop gestational diabetes (temporary diabetes occurring during pregnancy and generally clearing up after delivery), Dr. Jovanovic-Peterson gives guidance through the new challenges of testing blood sugar, eating to achieve normal blood sugars, taking insulin if necessary, safe exercise, labor, delivery, and breast-feeding.

Sweet Kids, by Betty Brackenridge, M.S., R.D., C.D.E. (1995) 60 min.

Betty's great depth of experience in counseling parents shows through clearly as she explains how to avoid food fights in the family. Trying to follow a diabetes meal plan can sometimes adversely impact the family relationships, especially when Mom and Dad become food police. You'll learn your job description as a parent and your child's job description as a diabetic as well. Using Betty's strategies will focus you on what counts and what doesn't in a diabetic child's eating plan. The result will be that your child's hunger will be satisfied and proper growth assured, and peace will reign at the dinner table.

FOR CHILDREN AND YOUNG PEOPLE

Baby-Sitters Club (a series of books for eight-to-twelve-year-old girls): *The Truth About Stacey* (1986, 167 pp.); *Stacey's Emergency* (1991, 147 pp.); *Stacey McGill, Super Sitter* (1996, 142 pp.), by Ann M. Martin.

Part of a popular series of novels about seven girls who run a baby-sitting service in their hometown. These three are about Stacy and her diabetes. "The Truth" is how she handles diabetes, and "Emergency" is when she gets overburdened with work and ends up in the hospital. "Super Sitter" is how she cares for an eight-year-old girl with diabetes. Very positive stories with accurate but nonintrusive diabetes information.

Donnie Makes a Difference, by Sandra Haines. (1994) 27 pp.

Donnie is a total football nut. He eats, sleeps, dreams, and, most important, plays football. Then he's tackled by diabetes and can't play. But he gets his diabetes under control and learns how to make a difference for his team and in everything he does. Colorful illustrations. For grades K through five.

In Control, by Jean Betschart, M.N., R.N., C.D.E., and Susan Thom, R.D., L.D., C.D.E. (1995) 125 pp.

The only (and much-needed!) self-help book for teens with diabetes. Talks teen language and tells true stories. Full of realistic problems and workable solutions. Covers all concerns, including birth control and sex, dating, parties and alcohol, career choice, parents and siblings, and above all, staying in control. Delightfully illustrated. Both authors got diabetes as teens themselves and have both become outstanding diabetes educators. Amazingly, both have been president of the AADE. What more can we say?

It's Time to Learn About Diabetes, by Jean Betschart, M.N., R.N., C.D.E. (Rev. 1995) 110 pp.

This workbook on diabetes for children ages eight to ten is creatively and professionally written by a highly experienced diabetes educator. Wonderfully illustrated. Fill-in quizzes for each chapter. A uniquely important book for home and diabetes class use. Invaluable for the newly diagnosed child.

COOKBOOKS: CONVENTIONAL
AND LOW-FAT

The Art of Cooking for the Diabetic, by Mary Abbott Hess, M.S., R.D., F.A.D.A. (3rd ed. 1997) 560 pp.

This brand-new edition of the best-selling classic has the latest ADA nutritional guidelines and 375 healthful and flavorsome recipes (low-cal, low-fat, high-fiber). It's the *Joy of Cooking* for the diabetic cuisine with half a million copies sold. Like having a master chef and a registered dietitian in your kitchen.

Diabetic Cookies, by Mary Jane Finsand. (1994) 160 pp.

This is a book for true Cookie Monster. Talk about variety—207 recipes; seventy-four drop cookies, seventy-five bar cookies, thirty-three shaped cookies, and twenty-five refrigerator cookies. Mainly sweetened with granulated sugar substitute and/or fructose. Easy, complete directions, nutritional analysis. Most cookies have only four grams of carbohydrate.

The Diabetic Sweet Tooth Cookbook, by Mary Jane Finsand. (1993) 159 pp.

A delectable array of cakes, frostings, cookies, candy, crepes, pies, ices and sherbets, drinks, sweet breads, and puddings. The last book Mary Jane wrote, and it includes her personal tips and tricks as well as invaluable conversion guides and recommended flavorings, extracts, herbs, and spices.

Free and EQUAL Cookbook, by Carole Kruppa. (2nd ed. 1994) 132 pp.

Update of the highly popular cookbook featuring dishes made with Equal (NutraSweet). The author grew up and learned her cooking in France, and it shows in the good taste of these 160 low-calorie and sugar-free recipes. Includes breakfast treats, appetizers, soups, salads, entrees, desserts, beverages, jams, and jellies. Calorie counts and exchanges for all recipes.

Free and EQUAL Dessert Cookbook, by Carole Kruppa. (1992) 167 pp.

Offers 150 quick and delicious low-calorie desserts and sweet treats, all using the sweetener Equal (NutraSweet) and all with the Carole Kruppa magic touch. These tasty treats are also low salt and low cholesterol. Exchanges and calories included.

The Joy of Snacks, by Nancy Cooper, R.D. (1991) 285 pp.

If you're a type 2, snacking six to ten times a day is actually better for you than three square meals. Type 1's need snacks to prevent or treat low-blood-sugar episodes. Here's the perfect book for both types by an acclaimed dietitian. Lots of muffin and cookie recipes and a large selection of popcorn treats and special snacks for kids. Two hundred great recipes in all, with exchanges.

Magic Menus for People with Diabetes, by the American Diabetes Association. (1996) 256 pp.

This book is similar to their previous *Month of Meals* series, only better, since it's all in one compact volume. Gives fifty different breakfasts, fifty lunches, seventy-five dinners, and thirty snacks. You can flip back and forth to any combination of breakfast, lunch, and dinner choices and the total calories will equal fifteen hundred (levels can be adjusted up or down to suit individual needs). Forget figuring fats, calories, and exchanges. It's all done for you automatically—it's truly like magic.

Quick and Delicious Diabetic Desserts, by Mary Jane Finsand. (1992) 190 pp.

Scores of recipes for pies and puddings, cakes and cookies, ice cream and tortes. No meal is complete without one of these luscious treats. Exchanges given.

Vegetarian Cooking for People with Diabetes, by Patricia LeShane. (Rev. and expanded 1994) 143 pp.

Over one hundred true vegan recipes without dairy products or eggs, emphasizing low-fat cooking. Soy milk, nuts, grains, and legumes used for protein. Sweeteners are small amounts of blackstrap molasses or honey. Sample dishes: grainburgers, millet with tofu and mushrooms, soybean mushroom pilaf, apple-oat drop cookies, and rice pudding. The recipes are easy to prepare, with exchanges and fat percentages given for each.

COOKBOOKS: LOW-CARBOHYDRATE DIET

Dr. Atkins New Diet Cookbook, by Robert C. Atkins, M.D., and Fran Gare, M.S. (1994) 248 pp.

Over two hundred of the most asked-for recipes at the Atkins Center for Complementary Medicine in New York City. They appear nondietetic because they are not fat restricted—the fat content is not even included—but they are carbohydrate restricted. There are seven kinds of hamburgers and other high-protein recipes such as roast turkey with almond stuffing and tuna meat loaf. Desserts include cheesecake, brownies, chocolate sponge layer cake, and coconut cream pie.

Dr. Atkins' Quick and Easy New Diet Cookbook, by Robert C. Atkins, M.D., and Veronica Atkins. (1997) 213 pp.

In this low-carbohydrate cookbook, Dr. Atkins' Russian-born wife, who's lived in seven countries, brings an international flare to the diet, including pleasurable desserts like Shortcake Veronique with a Kiss of Rum. A total of 160 recipes, with carbohydrate analysis. Tips for modifying other recipes to low-carbohydrate dining. Spiral bound.

The Low-Carb Cookbook, by Fran McCullough. (1998) 384 pp.

In this cookbook Fran McCullough takes the foods you *can* eat and makes them into something you *want to* eat, bringing her years of experience as a cookbook writer and editor to this ideal low-carb guide. Here are over 250 recipes with tips and cooking techniques to give you inspiration galore. Among your first strategies will be to throw out of your cupboard "virtually anything labeled low fat." Includes sweeteners and how to use them most effectively, what to drink, how to cope with entertaining and holidays, sources of low-carb products, and how to deal with plateaus.

FOOD GUIDES AND
NUTRITIONAL ANALYSIS

The Carbohydrate Addict's Gram Counter, by Richard F. Heller, Ph.D., and Rachael F. Heller, Ph.D. (1993) 90 pp.

The authors are both professors at Mt. Sinai School of Medicine in New York City. This comprehensive guide gives the calorie, fat, and carbohydrate counts for twenty-seven hundred foods, including many brand names. It also gives an analysis of menu items from fourteen fast-food chains. It indicates items that are low fat and heart healthy. Very accurate—the information was supplied by the U.S. Department of Agriculture, the U.S. Center for Disease Control, and other authoritative sources. Easy to use and carry in your pocket or purse as it's only six inches by four inches.

Carbohydrate Calories and Fat in Your Food, by Art Ulene, M.D. (1995) 682 pp.

No matter what you count, be it calories, carbohydrates, or fats, this is your master reference guide—thirty thousand entries in a brand-new edition. Easy to use. Includes brand-name and specialty foods, low-fat foods, and snacks. Over forty different kinds of peanut butter alone!

Convenience Food Facts, by Arlene Monk, R.D. (Rev. expanded ed. 1997) 456 pp.

A humdinger of a reference book. Tells all you need to know about everything in your grocery cart—calories, carbohydrate, fat, cholesterol, sodium, and exchanges. Over three thousand popular brand-name products, plus diabetically oriented ones like Estee.

Exchanges for All Occasions, by Marion Franz, M.S., R.D., C.D.E. (4th ed. 1997) 384 pp.

Your Guide to Choosing Healthy Food Anytime, Anywhere. Never has so much sound, authoritative guidance for diabetes eating been packed into one book. The latest nutritional facts and recommendations, including carbohydrate counting. Covers every eating situation and most cuisines (Jewish, Southwestern, vegetarian, etc.). Includes sample menus and twenty-nine recipes.

Fast Food Facts, by Marion Franz, R.D. (4th ed. 1994) 182 pp.

A pocket-size guide (4″ × 6″) for making the right food choices at fast-food restaurants. Complete nutritional information on over fifteen hundred menu offerings from the fifteen largest fast-food chains. Symbols designate items high in salt, fat, or sugar.

The Restaurant Companion, by Hope S. Warshaw, R.D. (2nd ed. 1995) 360 pp.

Focuses on restaurant dining, showing how to make healthy choices for seven kinds of ethnic cuisines (Mexican, Chinese, Italian, Thai, etc.), as well as vegetarian style, and American and fast-food restaurants. Advice for handling salad bars, pizza places, brunches, and airline meals.

AUDIO CASSETTES

Carbohydrate Counting, by Betty Brackenridge, M.S., R.D., C.D.E. (1995) 60 min.

Describes this increasingly popular system of meal planning that gives you more mealtime freedom and better control. Reveals how in spite of its simplicity, just counting grams of carbohydrates can help you zero in on the good diabetes control that may have been eluding you. The rationale is that carbohydrates (sugars and starches) have a much greater effect on blood sugar than protein and fat. Counting carbohydrates will show those of you who are "playing pancreas" with numerous insulin injections how to adjust your doses to the carbohydrates you eat. The system also works for type 2's by helping them match their food to their bodies' ability to produce insulin. Covers food label–reading, measuring portions, gram counting books, and adapting the exchange system to carbohydrate counting.

New Nutritional Guidelines, by Betty Brackenridge, M.S., R.D., C.D.E. (1995) 60 min.

If you're confused by the big changes in diet for diabetics announced in the 1994 ADA guidelines, here's help. Dietitian Betty Brackenridge answers the most commonly asked questions, such as: "What do you mean there's no more diabetic diet?" "What do you mean I can eat sugar?" "What do you mean I don't need to be my 'ideal weight'? " The 1994 guidelines are far more user friendly than the old and will bring back dining pleasures you thought were gone forever.

MAGAZINES

Countdown, 432 Park Avenue South, New York, NY 10016-8013 (1-800-223-1138). The magazine of the Juvenile Diabetes Foundation International. Published four times a year. Subscription price $25.

Diabetes Dateline, a publication of the National Diabetes Information Clearinghouse (NDIC), Bethesda, MD 20892-3560 (1-301-654-3327). Meant primarily for professionals but also contains up-to-date information of value to the diabetic population. Published two or three times a year. Subscription is free.

Diabetes Forecast, the magazine of the American Diabetes Association, 1660 Duke St., Alexandria, VA 22314 (1-800-232-3472). Published monthly. Membership dues are $24 per year, $10 of which is designated for the subscription.

Diabetes Interview, 3715 Balboa Street, San Francisco, CA 94121 (1-800-488-8468). A consumer-oriented newspaper for the diabetes community; includes reports on current research, business briefs, articles. Published monthly. Subscription price $14.

Diabetes Self-Management, P.O. Box 52890, Boulder, CO 80322-2890 (1-800-234-0923). A distinguished board of contributing editors provides articles of special usefulness for diabetes self-care. Published bimonthly. Subscription price $18.

The Diabetic Reader, June and Barbara, Ink/Prana Publications, 5623 Matilija Ave., Van Nuys, CA 91401 (1-800-735-7726). Reviews and excerpts latest books on diabetes, includes offbeat feature articles on living the good life with diabetes, catalog of available diabetes books and products. Published semiannually. Subscription price is $5.00 per year, $15 forever; sample copy free.

Index

About the Authors

June Biermann (diabetic for thirty-one years) and Barbara Toohey are the authors of nine books on diabetes, including *The Diabetic Woman* and *The Diabetic's Total Health Book*. They are codirectors of Prana Publications in Van Nuys, California, publisher of *The Diabetic Reader,* a semiannual newsletter promoting good health, good food, and good times for people with diabetes.